THE NON-MERIDIAL POINTS OF ACUPUNCTURE

The first book for professional acupuncturists to be devoted entirely to non-meridial points. The anatomical position of every point is both described and shown on the charts, the symptomatology of every point is given, and there is a full repertory for their use.

By the same author:
ACUPUNCTURE ATLAS AND REFERENCE BOOK
ACUPUNCTURE TREATMENT OF MUSCULO-SKELETAL CONDITIONS
CELESTIAL STEMS
MOXIBUSTION (co-authored with Roger Newman Turner)
SECONDARY VESSELS OF ACUPUNCTURE

THE NON-MERIDIAL POINTS OF ACUPUNCTURE

by

Royston Low
Ph.D., N.D., D.O., M.B.N.O.A., F.B.Ac.A., DrAc.

Illustrated by
Peter Cox and Stephen Lee

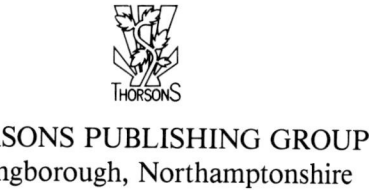

THORSONS PUBLISHING GROUP
Wellingborough, Northamptonshire

First published 1988

To my Wife, Eunice,
to my sons,
Ian and Christopher,
but also to
Dr Joshua Guan Dao Le,
who is using these points to
such good effect in the British
College of Acupuncture Teaching
Clinic.

© ROYSTON LOW 1988

All rights reserved. No part of this book may be reproduced or utilized in any form or by any means, electronic or mechanical, including photocopying, recording or by any information storage and retrieval system, without permission in writing from the Publisher.

British Library Cataloguing in Publication Data

Low, Royston H.
The non-meridial points of acupuncture.
1. Acupuncture
I. Title
615.8'92   RM184

ISBN 0-7225-1483-2

Published by Thorsons Publishers Limited, Wellingborough, Northamptonshire, NN8 2RQ, England

Printed in Great Britain by Woolnough Bookbinding, Irthlingborough, Northamptonshire

1 3 5 7 9 10 8 6 4 2

CONTENTS

Introduction	7
Special Points: Face	10
Head and Neck	13
Chest and Abdomen	16
Dorsal and Lumbar	19
Arm and Hand	22
Leg and Foot	25
Other Non-Meridial Points: Face (and Mouth)	30
Head and Neck	36
Chest and Abdomen	42
Dorsal and Lumbar	46
Arm and Hand	53
Leg and Foot	60
Hand Needling	71
Foot Needling	77
Nose and Face Needling	85
Head Needling	92
Kou Liang Techniques and Collective Loci	96
Repertory	99
General and Infectious Conditions	99
Endocrine Glands	100
Neurological Conditions	100
Brain	101
Mental Conditions	101
Musculo-Skeletal	102
Headaches	103

Sinusitis, Rhinitis etc.	103
Respiratory Tract	103
Circulatory	103
Genito-Urinary Tract	104
Gastro-Intestinal Disorders	104
Liver, Gall Bladder, Spleen and Pancreas	105
Gynaecology and Obstetrics	106
Male Sexual Disorders	106
Skin and Dermatology	106
Sense Organs	107
Cross-Index of Points	109

INTRODUCTION

I have actually heard one or two 'traditional' acupuncturists decry the use of non-meridial points on the grounds that they are not 'holistic' — treating a specific symptom rather than the patient as a whole!

Such a viewpoint is, of course, completely indefensible. Some of the non-meridial points, such as Yintang and Taiyang, are amongst the most important in the body, whilst Dannangxue is capable of having a stronger specific effect upon the gall-bladder as such than any other point. As in everything else, idealism needs to be tempered with knowledge and experience, and the more experienced the practitioner becomes the more he will find that he is embodying the non-meridial points into his naturally holistic prescriptions.

The reason for my writing this book is that I felt the need for a ready description of where the non-meridial points are and what they do — some charts give some of them, some charts give others, none of them give them all, and those that do show quite a few give them mingled with the normal points which, although useful for showing their relative positions, usually have so many points on view that it is often difficult to pick out the right one without considerable checking.

The usual greatest point of controversy is the system of numbering. Students complain piteously that Bensky calls Taiyang M-HN-9 whilst the Shanghai charts call it EM3 (and now I'm going to call it FA3!). The fact is that every book-writer and chart-maker uses his own system, and students will simply have to get used to learning enough Chinese to use the original name if they want to communicate with their fellows.

Writing up notes is another matter — it is far easier to write DL8 than Shiqizhui, and as long as practitioners stick to the one system and know to which points they are referring there should be no problem — unless someone else tries to find out what treatment was used!

For the purpose of this book I have divided the points up into the usual anatomical arrangement and split them up into two groups. Candidly, there are so many of them (and more are being discovered every day) that to put them all onto one set of charts would make quick referral impossible. I have therefore picked out the special ones, which everyone is using every day, and placed them in the first set. These I have called 'Special Points', and have numbered them:

Face	FA
Head and Neck	HN
Chest and Abdomen	CA
Dorsal and Lumbar	DL
Arm and Hand	AR
Leg and Foot	LE

The remaining points, to a considerable number, are appropriately called 'Other non-meridial points', and are numbered by the simple process of putting 'O' for 'Other' in front of the previous letters. By this means it will be immediately apparent as to whether the point is one of the most used ones or not, and also the charts will be far less 'cluttered' than would otherwise be the case.

I have endeavoured to include every known point, and have also included pages on Hand and Foot needling. These again are special points which can have very strong and specific effects, and their study by all practitioners is very seriously recommended. I have included head needling because, again, this is a technique of the greatest possible value.

Finally, the book concludes with a few notes on Kou Liang techniques and Collective Loci. These are not non-meridial points as such, as most of them are based upon the standard points, but they are combinations to which I feel the practitioner's attention should be peculiarly and forcibly directed. Most useful of all, of course, is the Repertory. I believe that this is the first time that the non-meridial points have been properly repertorized, and it is hoped this will prove a valuable addition to the practitioner's armamentarium.

SPECIAL POINTS

Special Points
FACE

FA1	Yintang ('Seal Hall')		Midway between the medial ends of the eye-brows, on the glabella.
		Insertion:	Slanting 3-5fen, either downwards or towards Bl2 (Zanzhu).
		Indications:	Headache, vertigo, rhinitis, hypertension, insomnia, infantile convulsions.
FA2	Yuyao ('Fish Waist')		In the hollow in the middle of the eye-brow, vertically above the pupil.
		Insertion:	Horizontal 2-5 fen, towards either Bl2 (Zanzhu) or TH23 (Sizhukong).
		Indications:	Supraorbital neuralgia; acute conjunctivitis; frontal sinusitis; cataract.
FA3	Taiyang ('Sun')		On the temple, in the depression 1 cun posterior to the mid-point between the external canthus and the tip of the eye-brow.
		Insertion:	Either perpendicular ½-1 cun or (for migraine) transverse to GB8 (Shuaigu) or (for facial paralysis) downwards to St6 (Jiache).
		Indications:	Headaches (lateral or vertex); migraine; sore red and swollen eyes.
FA4	Qiuhou ('Behind the Ball')		At the junction of the outer ¼ and the inner ¾ of the inferior border of the orbit.
		Insertion:	Vertical, into orbit, slightly medial and upwards, ½-1½ cun.
		Indications:	Glaucoma; myopia; inflammation or atrophy of optic nerve; retinitis pigmentosa; convergent squint; cataract.
FA5	Shangming ('Upper Brightness')		Directly below Yuyao, beneath superior border of the orbit.
		Insertion:	Vertical, along upper border of orbit, 1-1½ cun.
		Indications:	Atrophy of optic nerve; ametropia; keratoleukoma.
FA6	Waiming ('Outer Brightness')		3 fen above external canthus.
		Insertion:	Vertical, along upper border of orbit, 1-1½ cun.
		Indications:	Atrophy of optic nerve; ametropia; keratoleukoma.
FA7	Shangyingxian ('Upper Welcome Fragrance')		5 fen below internal canthus.
		Insertion:	Downwards along side of nose, 3-5 fen.
		Indications:	Rhinitis; nasal polypii; nasosinusitis.

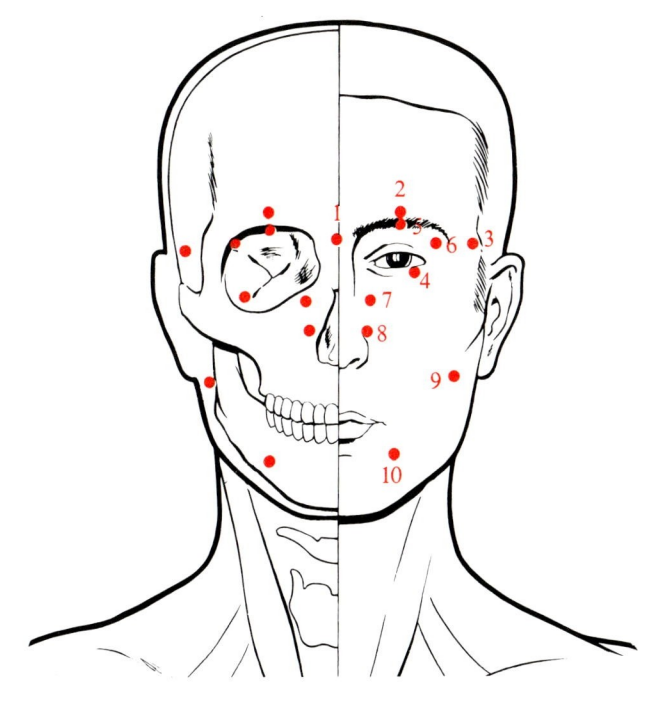
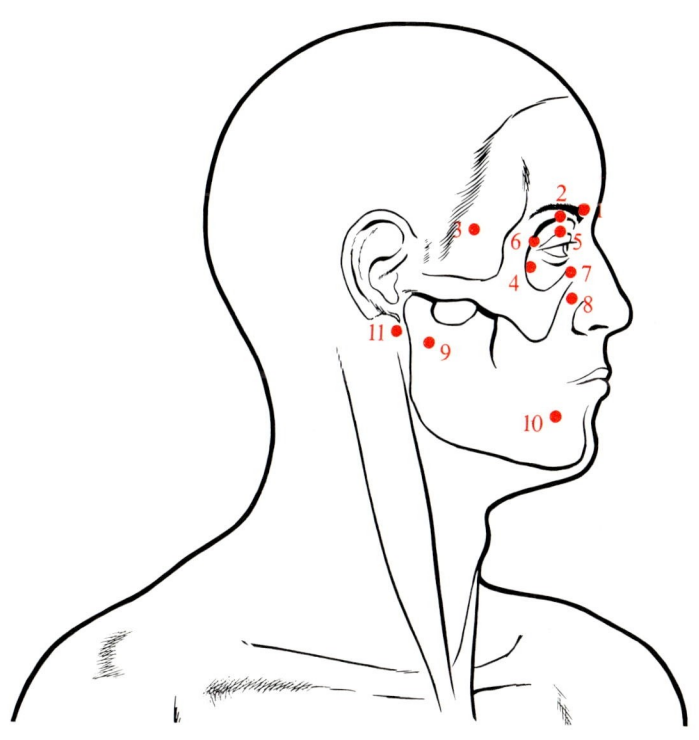

11

FA8	Bitong ('Nose Passage')	Insertion:	In depression below nasal bone, at the upper end of the nasolabial sulcus. Either slanting upwards towards bridge of nose or downwards along side of nose, 3-6 fen.
		Indications:	Rhinitis; nasal polypii; nasosinusitis.
FA9	Qianzhong ('Pull Aright')	Insertion:	½-1 cun anterior to auditory meatus, in masseter muscle on buccal branch of facial nerve. Slanting forward ½-1 cun.
		Indications:	Facial paralysis; parotitis; mouth ulcers.
FA10	Jiachengjiang ('Grasping Contain Fluid') (Also known as *Keliou*).	Insertion:	Lateral to CV24 (Chengjiang), directly below St4 (Dicang), in the mental foramen. Vertical, 2-5 fen, *or* for trigeminal neuralgia into mental foramen and slant medial and downwards 5 fen.
		Indications:	Trigeminal neuralgia; facial paralysis or spasm.
FA11	Tingling ('Hearing's Inspiration')	Insertion:	¾ of the distance from SI19 (Tinggong) to GB2 (Tinghui). Vertical, 1½-2 cun (open mouth slightly).
		Indications:	Tinnitus; deafness; deaf-mutism.

Special Points
HEAD AND NECK

HN1	Yilong ('Shielding Deafness')	Insertion: Indications:	In depression 3 fen above TH17 (Yifeng), behind ear. Slanted, slightly forwards and downwards, 1 cun. Tinnitus; deafness; deaf-mutism.
HN2	Yiming ('Shielding Brightness')	Insertion: Indications:	1 cun posterior to TH17 (Yifeng). Vertical, ½-1 cun. Myopia; hypermetropia; night blindness; atrophy of optic nerve; cataract; tinnitus; vertigo; parotitis; headache; insomnia; mental illness.
HN3	Anmian 1 ('Peaceful Sleep')	Insertion: Indications:	Midway between Yiming and TH17. Vertical, 1½-2 cun. Insomnia; migraine; schizophrenia.
HN4	Anmian 2 ('Peaceful Sleep')	Insertion: Indications:	Midway between GB20 (Fengchi) and Yiming. Vertical, 1-2 cun. Insomnia; restlessness; palpitations; schizophrenia.
HN5	Biantao ('Tonsil')	Insertion: Indications:	Below lower border of angle of mandible, in front of carotid artery. Vertical, 1-1½ cun. Tonsillitis; pharyngitis.
HN6	Shanglianquan ('Upper Spring of Integrity')	Insertion: Indications:	1 cun above laryngeal prominence, in depression between mandible and hyoid bone. Slanting to root of tongue, 1-1½ cun. Slurred speech; mutism; salivation; acute or chronic pharyngitis; stomatitis.
HN7	Zengyin ('Increase Sound')	Insertion: Indications:	Midway between the laryngeal prominence and the angle of the mandible. Towards laryngopharynx, ½-1 cun. (Avoid carotid artery). Aphonia due to disease of vocal cords.
HN8	Xinshi ('New Recognition')	Insertion: Indications:	1½ cun lateral to lower end of spinous process of 3rd cervical. Vertical, ½-1 cun. Stiff neck; occipital headache; sore throat.
HN9	Bailao ('Hundred Labours')	Insertion: Indications:	1 cun lateral and ½ cun below lower end of spinous process of 3rd cervical. Vertical, ½-1 cun. Stiff neck; cough; scrofula.

HN10	Jingbi ('Neck and Arm')		⅓ distance from medial end of clavicle to its lateral end, up 1 cun, at posterior margin of sternocleidomastoid muscle.
		Insertion:	Vertical 5-8 fen. (Caution — Avoid needling downwards into apex of lung).
		Indications:	Numbness in arm; brachial neuralgia; paralysis of upper limb.

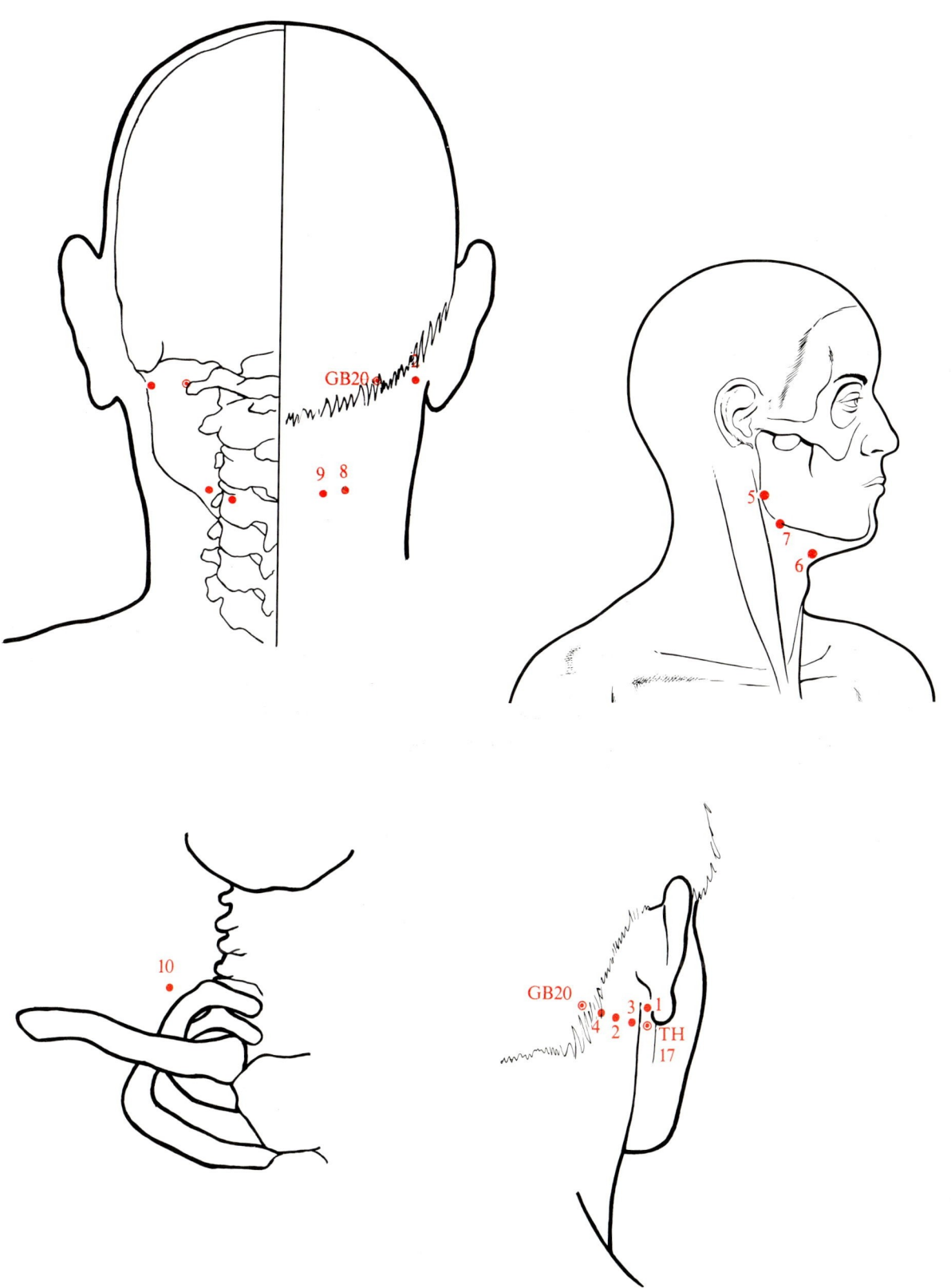

Special Points
CHEST AND ABDOMEN

CA1	Tiwei ('Lift Stomach')	Insertion: Indications:	4 cun lateral to CV12 (Zhongwan). Slant to St25 (Tianshu), 2-3 cun. Prolapsed stomach; indigestion.
CA2	Shuishang ('Above Water')	Insertion: Indications:	Midway between CV9 (Shuifen) and CV10 (Xiawan). Vertical, 1-1½ cun. Diarrhoea; abdominal pain or distension; gastric hyperacidity.
CA3	Weile ('Stomach's Happiness')	Insertion: Indications:	2 fen above and 4 cun lateral to CV9 (Shuifen). 8 fen below Weishangxue. Vertical, 1-1½ cun. Pain in gastric area; prolapse of stomach.
CA4	Weishangxue ('Above the Stomach Orifice')	Insertion: Indications:	4 cun lateral to CV10 (Xiawan). Transverse, either towards navel or to St25 (Tianshu) 1-2 cun. Prolapsed stomach; abdominal distension.
CA5	Xingqixue ('New Qi Orifice')	Insertion: Indications:	With the navel as the apex of an equilateral triangle, each side 3 cun long, this point is situated at either end of the base line. Vertical, ½-1 cun. Infertility; pelvic inflammatory conditions.
CA6	Tituoxue ('Lift and Support Orifice')	Insertion: Indications:	4 cun lateral to CV4 (Guanyuan). Vertical, 1-1½ cun. Prolapsed uterus; pain in lower abdomen; hernia.
CA7	Weibao ('Support Placenta')	Insertion: Indications:	In depression below and medial to the anterior superior iliac spine, approximately level with CV4 (Guanyuan). Slanted along inguinal ligament, 2-3 cun. Prolapsed uterus; hernia; intestinal dysfunction.
CA8	Zhixie ('Stop Diarrhoea')	Insertion: Indications:	Midway between CV5 (Shimen) and CV4 (Guanyuan). Vertical, 1-2 cun. Dysentery; enteritis; retention of urine; enuresis.
CA9	Zigong ('Uterus')	Insertion: Indications:	3 cun lateral to CV3 (Zhongji). Vertical, 1-2 cun, also moxa. Prolapsed uterus; dysmenorrhoea; irregular menses; pelveoperitonitis; female sterility; pyelonephritis; cystitis; orchitis; appendicitis.

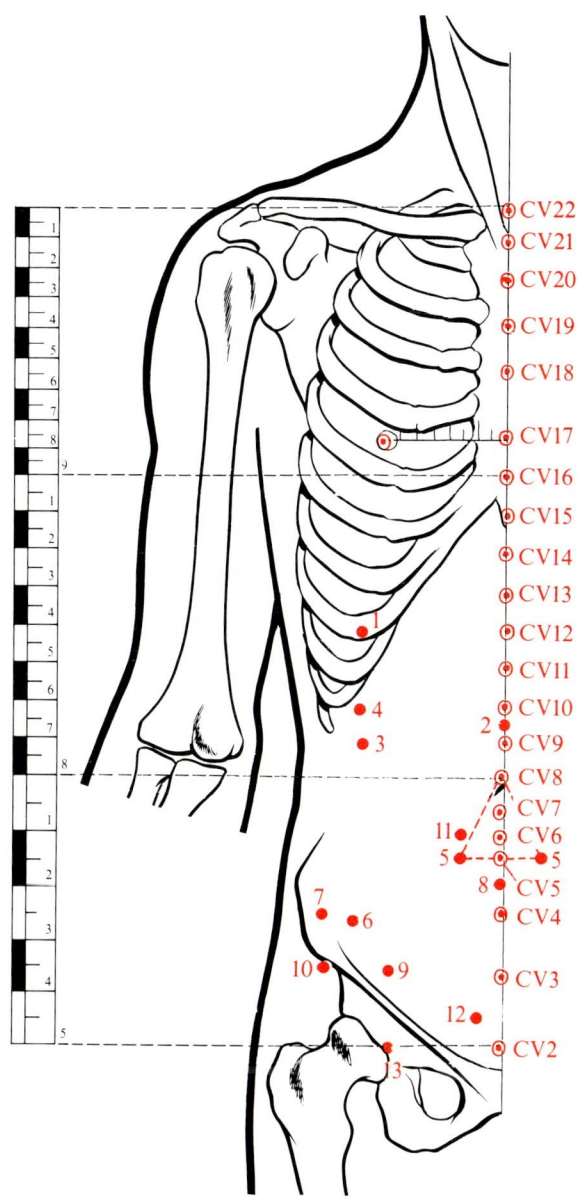

17

CA10	Shuxi ('Mouse Path')		Just under 6 cun lateral to CV3 (Zhongji). Approximately ⅓ length of inguinal ligament from its lateral end.
		Insertion:	Vertical, 1-2 cun.
		Indications:	Poor circulation in legs; weakness of leg adductors; TB of inguinal lymph glands.
CA11	Qizhong ('Middle of Qi')		1½ cun lateral to CV6 (Qihai).
		Insertion:	Vertical, 1½-2 cun.
		Indications:	Abdominal pain or distension; borborygmus; anaemia.
CA12	Yeniao ('Night Urine')		1 cun lateral to midway between CV2 (Qugu) and CV3 (Zhongji).
		Insertion:	Slanted, 1-1½ cun.
		Indications:	Bed-wetting.
CA13	Chongjian ('Pour Between')		3 cun lateral to CV2 (Qugu).
		Insertion:	Vertical, 1-2 cun.
		Indications:	Uterine prolapse; paralysis of legs.

Special Points
DORSAL AND LUMBAR

DL1	Huatuojiaji Points		A group of points on both sides of the spinal column at the lateral borders of each spinous process, about ½ cun lateral to the midline. They extend from C1 to S4, though some authorities limit them to D1 to L5 (Not illustrated).
		Insertion:	Slightly oblique towards midline, cervical and dorsal ½-1 cun, lumbar ½-2 cun. Can also use moxa.
		Indications:	Rather similar to Back-Shu points. C1-4 — diseases of the head region; C1-7 — diseases of the neck region; C3-D7 — diseases of the upper extremities; D1-7 — diseases of the thoracic area; D8-12 — diseases of the abdominal area; D10-L5 —diseases of the lumbar region; L2-S2 — diseases of the lower extremities; S1-4 — urogenital disorders. May also be used to treat local muscular conditions.
	(a) Chisanxue		— 3 special loci, Jiaji points lateral to GV15 (Yamen), D2 and L2, used for spondylitis, spinal meningitis and diseases of the spinal cord.
	(b) Xutse		— Lateral to D3 spine: Bronchitis, pleuritis, pneumonia; back-pain.
DL2	Xueyadian ('Blood Pressure Points')		2 cun lateral to lower end of spinous process of C6.
		Insertion:	Vertical, ½-1 cun.
		Indications:	High or low blood-pressure.
DL3	Dingchuan ('Stop Wheezing')		½ cun lateral to GV14 (Dazhuei).
		Insertion:	Oblique to vertebral body ½-1 cun, or moxa.
		Indications:	Asthma; cough; stiff neck; pain in shoulder and back.
DL4	Jiantongdian ('Shoulder Pain Point')		Middle of lateral border of scapula.
		Insertion:	Vertical, ½-¾ cun.
		Indications:	Shoulder joint problems. Paresis in upper limb.
DL5	Weishu ('Stomach's Comfort')		4½ cun lateral to L2, at intersection of 12th rib and sacro-spinalis muscle.
		Insertion:	Vertical, 1-2 cun.
		Indications:	Pain or spasm in stomach; gastric ulcer.
DL6	Shenzi ('Kidney Spine')		½ cun lateral to lower end of L2 spine. Jiaji point.
		Insertion:	Vertical, 1½-2 cun.
		Indications:	Spondylitis; inflammation of vertebral ligaments; paralysis of lower limb.

DL7	Yaoyan ('Waist's Eye')		On outer bladder line, lateral to spinous process of L3, below Bl47 (Zhishi), at lateral margin of sacro-spinalis muscle.
		Insertion:	Vertical, 1-2 cun.
		Indications:	Lumbago; gynaecological conditions.
DL8	Shiqizhui ('Below 17 Vertebrae')		Below spinous process of L5.
		Insertion:	Vertical, 1-1½ cun. Can use moxa or heated needle.
		Indications:	Pain lumbo-sacral area; sciatica; menstrual disorders; traumatic paraplegia.
DL9	Yaoqi ('Lower Back's Miscellany')		Below S2 spine.
		Insertion:	Slanted upwards, 2-2½ cun.
		Indications:	Epilepsy.
DL10	Huanzhong ('Circle's Middle')		Middle of a line connecting GB30 (Huantiao) and GV2 (Yaoshu).
		Insertion:	Vertical 2-3 cun.
		Indications:	Sciatica; lumbago.
DL11	Wuming ('5 Brightnesses')		In depression below spinous process of D2. (Locate with neck bent).
		Insertion:	Obliquely upwards, ½-1 cun.
		Indications:	Mania.

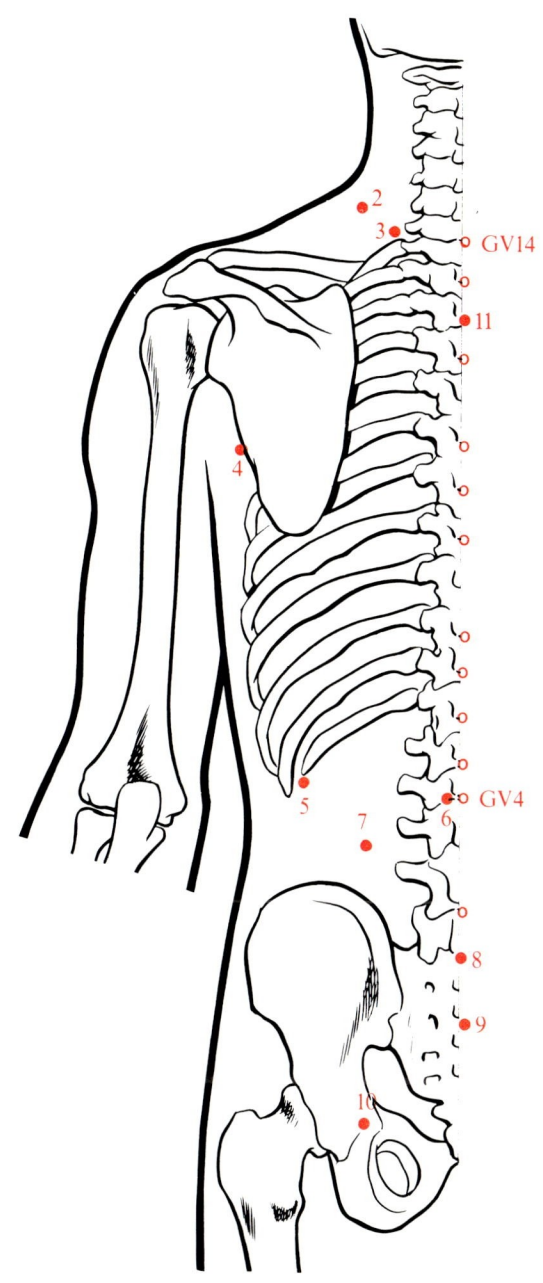

Special Points
ARM AND HAND

AR1	Jianneiling ('Shoulder's Inner Tomb')		With arm hanging at side, midway between Co15 (Jianyu) and the top of the anterior axillary crease.
		Insertion:	Vertical, to back of shoulder, ½-1 cun. For tendosynovitis of long head of biceps, slanted 2-3 cun.
		Indications:	Pain in shoulder joint; hemiplegia; hypertension; excessive sweating.
AR2	Jianqian (Chien-Chien)		1 cun above top of anterior axillary crease.
		Insertion:	Vertical, 1 cun.
		Indications:	Pain and stiffness in shoulder.
AR3	Taijian ('Lift Shoulder')		Midway between Co15 (Jianyu) and Lu1 (Zhongfu).
		Insertion:	Vertical, 1 cun.
		Indications:	Pain and stiffness in shoulder. After-effects of poliomyelitis.
AR4	Jubi ('Raise Arm')		2 cun below Taijian.
		Insertion:	Vertical, 1-1½ cun.
		Indications:	After-effects of poliomyelitis.
AR5	Naoshang ('Above the Scapula')		In the middle of the deltoid muscle.
		Insertion:	Vertical, 1-2 cun.
		Indications:	Upper limb hemiplegia; pain in shoulder and arm.
AR6	Gongzhong ('Middle of Humerus')		2½ cun below HC2 (Tianquan), on upper arm.
		Insertion:	Vertical, 1-1½ cun.
		Indications:	Paralysis of upper limb; inability to raise arm; wrist-drop; palpitations.
AR7	Bizhong ('Middle of Arm')		At midpoint between transverse creases of wrist and elbow, between radius and ulna, 1 cun proximal to HC4 (Ximen).
		Insertion:	Straight through the arm (through interosseous membrane) but not penetrating the skin on the opposite side.
		Indications:	Hemiplegia; spasms of upper limb; neuralgia of forearm; hysteria.
AR8	Jianhao ('Right Shoulder')		1½ cun above posterior axillary crease. About 8 fen above S19 (Jianzhen).
		Insertion:	Vertical, 1-1½ cun.
		Indications:	Stiffness in shoulder joint.
AR9	Yingshang ('Above the Olecranon')		4 cun above the olecranon of the elbow.
		Insertion:	Vertical, ½-1 cun.
		Indications:	Sequelae of poliomyelitis; palpitations.

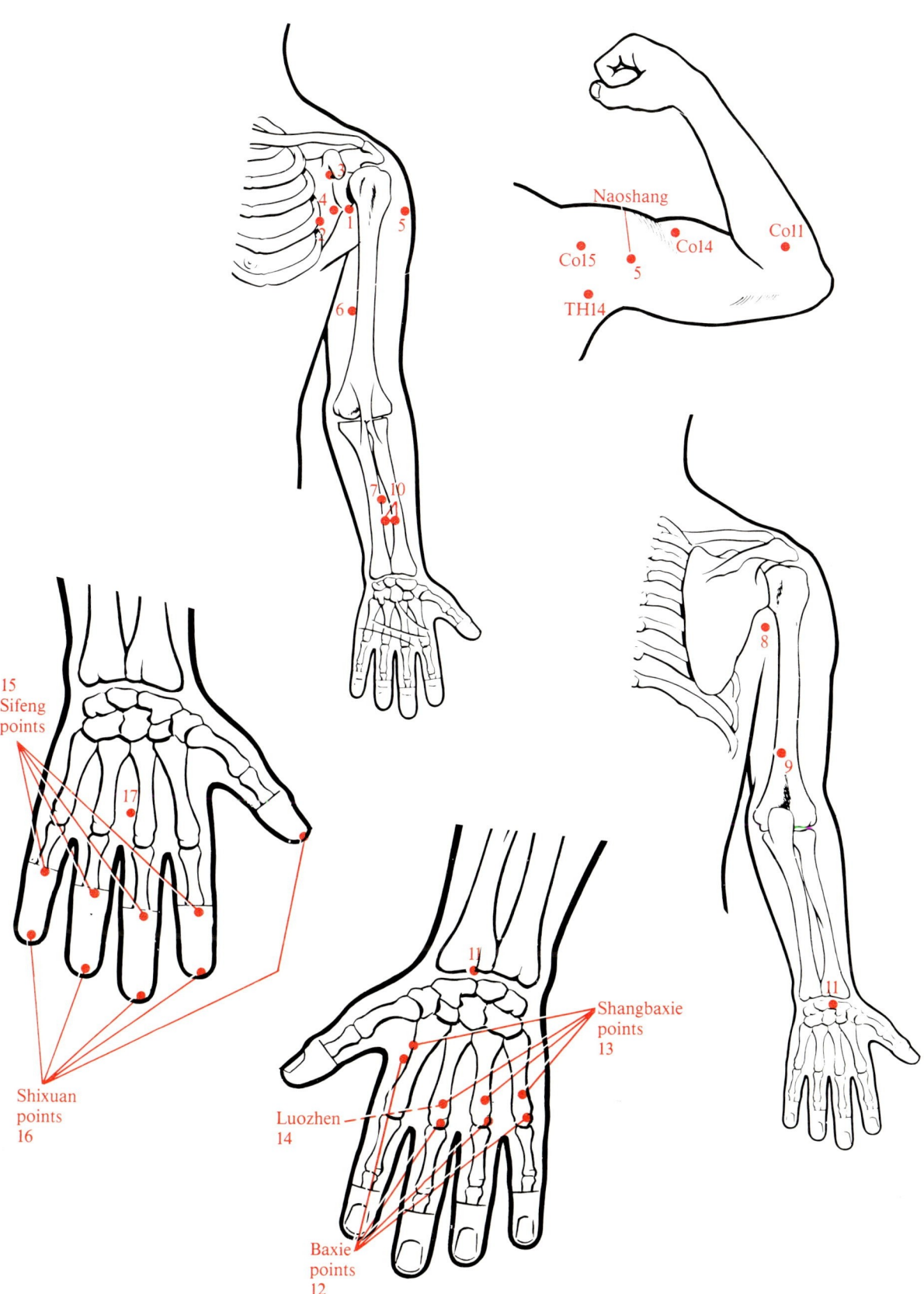

AR10	Erbai ('Two Whites')		4 cun proximal to wrist crease — two points, one between the two tendons, the other on the radial side of the tendons.
		Insertion:	Vertical, ½-1 cun.
		Indications:	Neuralgia of forearm; haemorrhoids; anal prolapse.
AR11	Zhongquan ('Middle Spring')		In depression on dorsum of wrist, between Co5 (Yangxi) and TH4 (Yangchi).
		Insertion:	Vertical, 3-5 fen.
		Indications:	Bronchitis; asthma; gastralgia; conditions of wrist and local tissues.
AR12	Baxie points ('Eight Evils')		Between the heads of each of the metacarpal bones — 4 on each hand. Insert with the hand formed into a fist.
		Insertion:	Straight along metacarpal bone, up to 1 cun.
		Indications:	Diseases of finger joints; numbness in fingers; stiff neck; headache; sore throat; toothache.
AR13	Shangbaxie ('Upper Eight Evils')		4 points on each hand, in the small depression just behind and between the metacarpophalangeal joints on the dorsum. (Two of these are Co4 (Hegu) and TH3 (Zhongzhu), and one is Luozhen.)
		Insertion:	Vertical, 3-5 fen.
		Indications:	As Baxie points.
AR14	Luozhen ('Stiff Neck')		½ cun behind and between the 2nd and 3rd metacarpophalangeal joints on the dorsum of the hand.
		Insertion:	Vertical or slanted, ½-1 cun.
		Indications:	Stiff neck; migraine; sore throat; stomach ache; pain in shoulder and arm.
AR15	Sifeng ('Four Seams')		On palmar surface of each finger, in centre of proximal interphalangeal crease.
		Insertion:	Prick, to draw a small amount of serum.
		Indications:	Arthritis of fingers; pertussis; infantile indigestion; faulty assimilation in infants.
AR16	Shixuan ('Ten Spreadings')		Ten points, one in the middle of each finger tip, about 1 fen from nail.
		Insertion:	Shallow insertion, or bleeding.
		Indications:	High fever; fainting; heat exhaustion; hysteria; numbness in finger tips.
AR17	Yatong ('Toothache')		On palmar surface, between 3rd and 4th metacarpal bones, 1 cun below metacarpophalangeal crease.
		Insertion:	Vertical, ½ cun.
		Indications:	Toothache.

Special Points
LEG AND FOOT

LE1	Zuogu ('Ischium')	Insertion: Indications:	1 cun below midpoint between coccyx and greater trochanter. Vertical; 2-3 cun. Sciatica; paralysis of leg.
LE2	Weiyinlian ('Outer Yin's Modesty')	Insertion: Indications:	One finger width below inguinal ligament, lateral to femoral artery, on the pulse. Vertical, slightly laterally, 1-1½ cun. (Care with artery). Paralysis of leg; pain low-back and leg; neuralgia of femoral nerve.
LE3	Maibu ('Stride')	Insertion: Indications:	6 cun below head of trochanter, on lateral margin of rectus femoris and vastus lateralis. Vertical, 1-2 cun. Hemiplegia; sequelae of poliomyelitis.
LE4	Heding ('Crane's Top')	Insertion: Indications:	In depression at the middle of the superior border of the patella. Vertical, ½ cun. Troubles with the knee joint and surrounding tissues.
LE5	Xiyan points ('Eyes of the Knee')	Insertion: Indications:	Below patella in hollow on either side of tendon. Lateral one is St35 (Dubi). With knee flexed, vertically 1-2 cun. Diseases of knee joint.
LE6	Lanweixue ('Appendix Orifice')	Insertion: Indications:	2 cun below St36 (Zusanli). Vertical, 1-1½ cun. Acute and chronic appendicitis; paralysis of leg; foot-drop; indigestion.
LE7	Dannangxue ('Gall Bladder Orifice')	Insertion: Indications:	1-2 cun below GB34 (Yanglingquan) between peroneus longus and extensor digitorum longus. Vertical, 1-1½ cun. Diseases of biliary duct; paralysis of lower limb.
LE8	Linghou ('Behind the Tomb')	Insertion: Indications:	Posterior to the head of the fibula, in a slight depression which feels numb and painful on pressure. Vertical, ½-1 cun. Sciatica; arthritis of knee; paralysis of lower limb.
LE9	Genjin ('Rigid Heel')	Insertion: Indications:	1½ cun below Bl57 (Chengshan). Vertical, 1 cun. Foot-drop and club-foot due to poliomyelitis.

LE10	Naoquing ('Brain's Clearing')	Insertion: Indications:	2 finger-widths above St41 (Jiexi), at lateral border of tibia. Vertical, ½-1 cun. Lassitude; vertigo; amnesia; mental retardation from encephalitis; foot-drop from poliomyelitis.
LE11	Genping ('Level with the Heel')	Insertion: Indications:	On the Achilles tendon, on a line connecting the medial and lateral malleoli. Vertical, 5-8 fen. Foot-drop and club-foot due to poliomyelitis.
LE12	Bafeng points ('Eight Winds')	Insertion: Indications:	In the web between each of the toes, four on each foot. 3 of these are Li2 (Xingjian), St44 (Neiting) and GB43 (Xiaxi). Slanted, ½-1 cun. Peripheral neuritis; inflammation of dorsum of foot and toes; headache; toothache; gastralgia; irregular menses.
LE13	Shangbafeng points ('Upper Eight Winds')	Insertion: Indications:	Posterior to the metatarsophalangeal joints of the toes, between all of the metatarsal bones. 3 of these are Li3 (Taichong), St43 (Xiangu) and GB42 (Diwuhui). Vertical, ½-1 cun. As for Bafeng points.

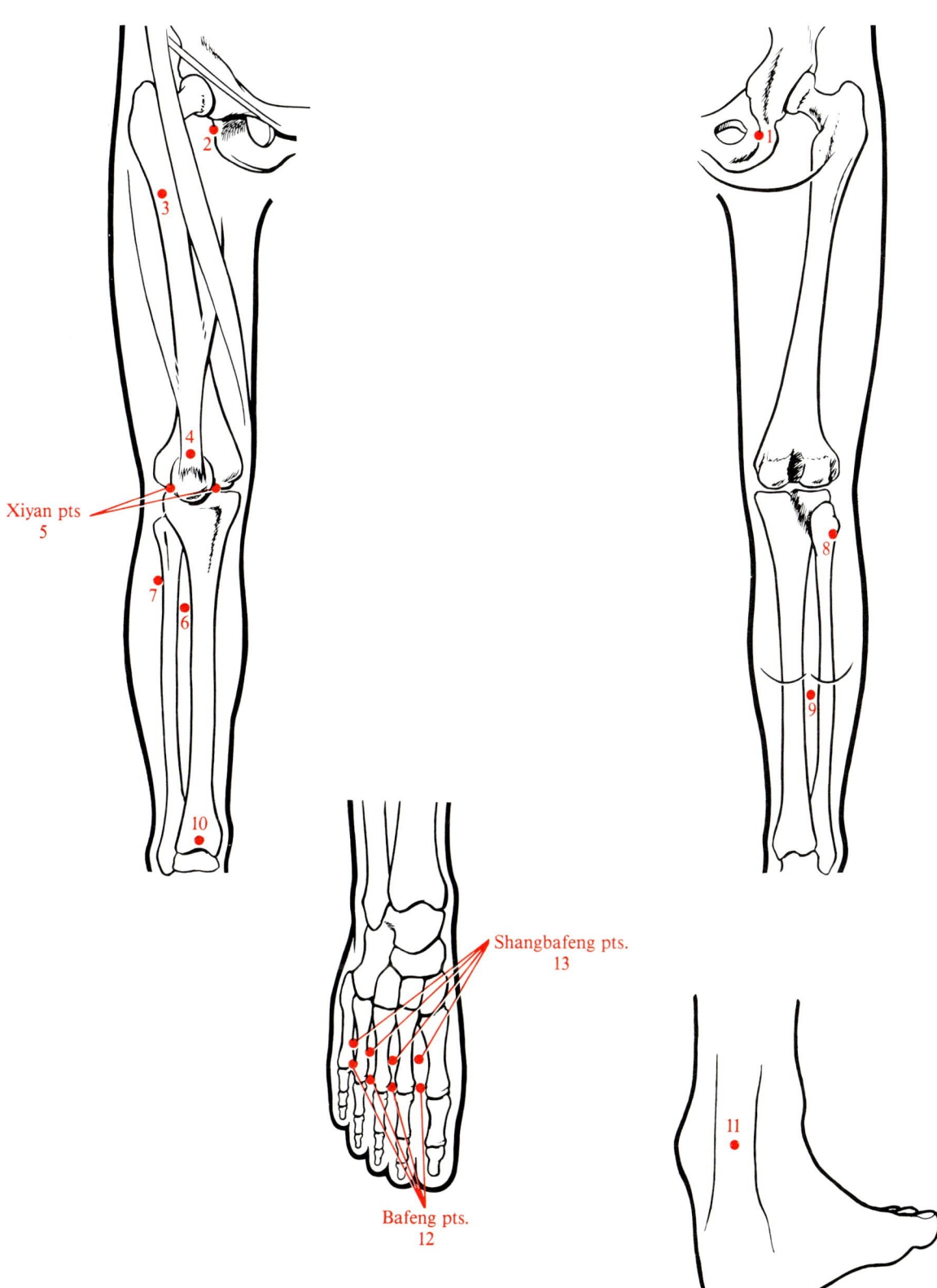

OTHER NON-MERIDIAL POINTS

Other Non-Meridial Points
FACE (AND MOUTH)

OFA1	Shangjingming ('Upper Eyes Bright')	Insertion: Indications:	2 fen superior to Bl1 (Jingming). Vertical, 1-1½ cun. Optic nerve atrophy; strabismus; ametropia; eyes water due to wind.
OFA2	Xiajingming ('Lower Eyes Bright')	Insertion: Indications:	2 fen below Bl1 (Jingming). Vertical, 1-1½ cun. As OFA1.
OFA3	Jianming ('Strengthens Brightness')	Insertion: Indications:	2 fen below and slightly lateral to OFA2, just inside the inferior margin of the orbit. Along the margin of the orbit, slightly towards the internal canthus, 1-1½ cun. Retinitis; retinitis pigmentosa; optic nerve atrophy; cataract; strabismus; ametropia; dacryocystitis.
OFA3a	Jianming 1 ('Strengthens Brightness')	Insertion: Indications:	Between Jianming and St1 (Chengqi), on medial side of the inferior margin of the orbit. As for Jianming. Corneal ulcer; nebula.
OFA3b	Jianming 2 ('Strengthens Brightness')	Insertion: Indications:	Between St1 (Chengqi) and FA4 (Qiuhou), inside the inferior margin of the orbit. As for Jianming. Optic nerve atrophy; nebula; retinochoroiditis; dacryocystitis; macula corneae.
OFA3c	Jianming 3 ('Strengthens Brightness')	Insertion: Indications:	3 fen lateral and superior to FA4 (Qiuhou), just inside the lateral margin of the orbit. As for Jianming. Optic nerve atrophy; strabismus.
OFA3d	Jianming 4 ('Strengthens Brightness')	Insertion: Indications:	3 fen above Shangjingming (OFA1), just inside the superior medial corner of the orbit. As for Jianming. Glaucoma; ametropia; cataract.
OFA4	Zengming 1 ('Increase Brightness')	Insertion: Indications:	2 fen medial to Shangming (FA5). Slightly towards internal canthus along the orbital margin. Nebula; cataract; ametropia.
OFA4a	Zengming 2 ('Increase Brightness')	Insertion: Indications:	2 fen lateral to Shangming (FA5). As for Zengming 1. As for Zengming 1.
OFA5	Neijingming ('Inner Eyes Bright')	Insertion: Indications:	Inner canthus of eye, just above lacrimal caruncle. Vertical, ½-1 cun. Retinal haemorrhage; optic nerve atrophy; conjunctivitis.

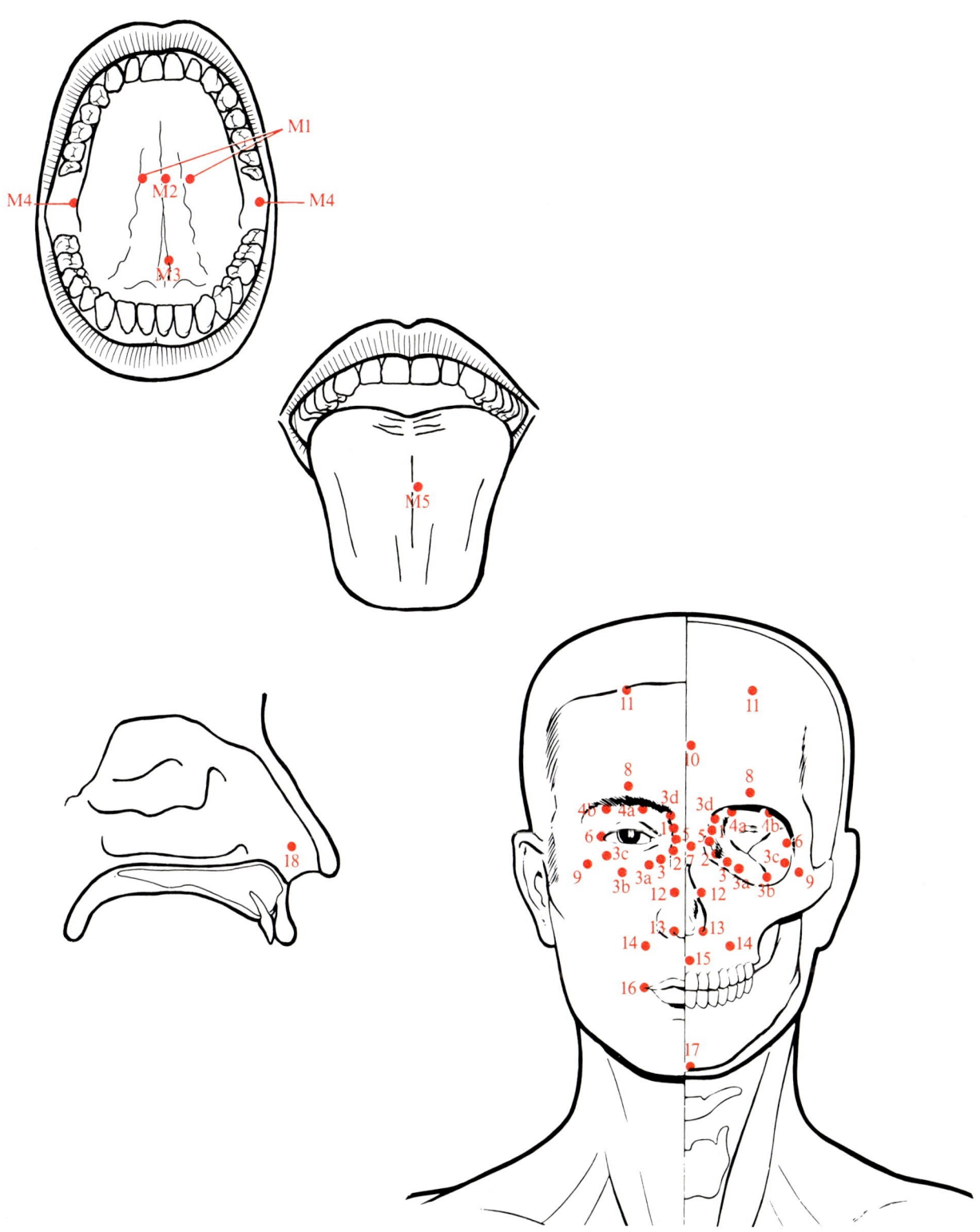

OFA6	Yuwei ('Fish-tail')	Insertion: Indications:	1 fen lateral to external canthus. Slanting, 2-5 fen. Eye diseases; facial paralysis; migraine.
OFA7	Shangen ('Mountain's Base')	Insertion: Indications:	Midway between the internal canthii of the eyes, on the bridge of the nose. Slanting, 3-5 fen. Headache; dizziness; blurred vision; sinusitis.
OFA8	Touguangming ('Brightness on the Head')	Insertion: Indications:	Directly above pupil, on upper border of eye-brow. Slanting, 3-5 fen. Myopia; palpebritis; paralysis of eye muscles; migraine.
OFA9	Tongming ('Pupil's Brightness')	Insertion: Indications:	½ cun below GB1 (Tongziliao). Slanted, ½-1 cun. Ametropia.
OFA10	Ezhong (Forehead's Middle')	Insertion: Indications:	1 cun above Yintang (FA1). Slanted, ½-1 cun. Sinusitis; insomnia; vertigo; palpitations.
OFA11	Muming ('Vision Bright')	Insertion: Indications:	Vertically above pupil, on border of hair-line. ½ cun below GB15 (Linqi). Slanted, 5-8 fen. Headache; conjunctivitis; weak sight.
OFA12	Jiabi ('Cheek and Nose')	Insertion: Indications:	On border of nasal bone and nasal cartilage, superior and medial to Bitong (FA8). Slanting, 3-5 fen. Rhinitis; nasal furuncle.
OFA13	Biliu ('Runny Nose')	Insertion: Indications:	Outer nostril, on the line connecting the septum nasi and the ala nasi. Slanting, 3-5 fen. Rhinitis; hyposmia; trigeminal neuralgia; facial paralysis.
OFA14	Sanxiao ('Spread Smile')	Insertion: Indications:	In middle of naso-labial sulcus, below and posterior to Co20 (Ying xian). Slanting, 3-5 fen. Rhinitis; nasal furuncle; facial paralysis.
OFA15	Dingshen ('Little Spirit')	Insertion: Indications:	Below GV26 (Renzhong), in philtrum ⅓ distance from top of lip to base of nose. Slanting upwards ½-1 cun. Psychosis; fits; dysmenorrhoea.
OFA16	Yankou ('Swallow's Mouth')	Insertion: Indications:	At the corner of the mouth, on the border between lips and cheek. Slanted, 5-8 fen. Trigeminal neuralgia; facial paralysis; constipation; urinary retention.
OFA17	Dihe ('Earth's Union')	Insertion: Indications:	The most prominent part on the midline of the mandible. Slanted, 2-3 fen. Pain in lower teeth; facial paralysis.

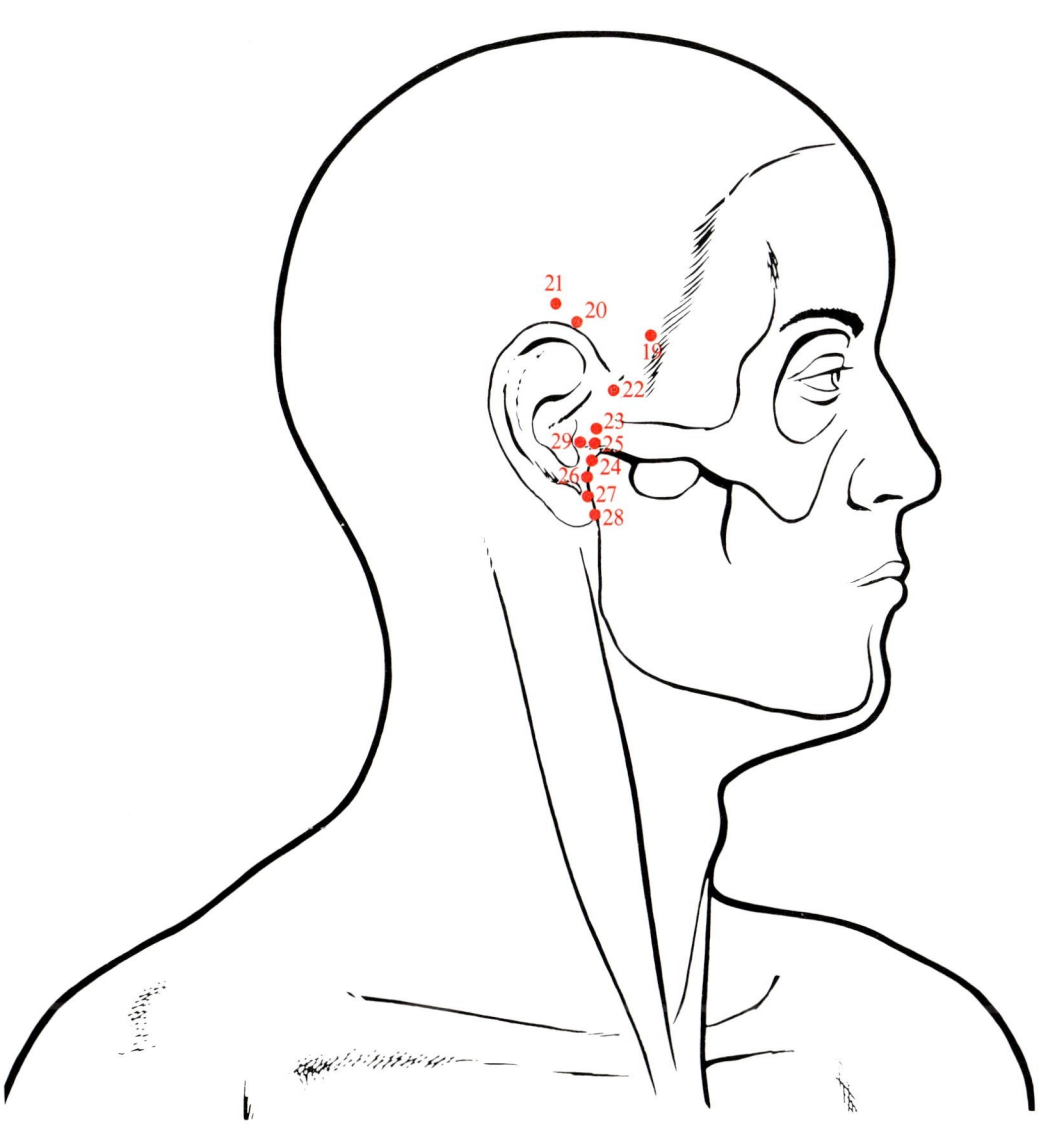

OFA18	Neiyingxiang ('Inner Welcome Fragrance')	Insertion: Indications:	Near the nostril opening in the mucous membrane on the nasal septum. Bleed. Conjunctivitis; laryngitis; heat-stroke.
OFA19	Tounie ('Temple')	Insertion: Indications:	1 cun posterior to Taiyang (FA3), level with the tip of the ear. (At a prominence in the temporal region on clenching the teeth.) Slanted, 1-1½ cun. Psychosis; fits; progressive loss of memory.
OFA20	Ehrjian ('Ear Tip')	Insertion: Indications:	At the tip of the auricle when the ear is bent forward. Vertical, 1-2 fen, or bleed. Conjunctivitis; migraine; cataract.
OFA21	Guangcai ('Lustre')	Insertion: Indications:	In a small depression 2 fen above and 1 fen anterior to the tip of the ear. Moxa (peck with green-stick). Infectious parotitis.
OFA22	Tingxiang ('Hear Sound')	Insertion: Indications:	1 fen above TH21 (Ermen), in small hollow. Vertical, ½-1 cun. Deafness.
OFA23	Shanglong ('Upper Deafness')	Insertion: Indications:	Midway between TH21 (Ermen) and SI19 (Tinggong). Vertical, 1-2 cun, with mouth open. Deafness; deaf-mutism.
OFA24	Tingxue ('Hearing Orifice')	Insertion: Indications:	Midway between SI19 (Tinggong) and GB2 (Tinghui). Vertical, 1-2 cun, with mouth open. Deaf-mutism.
OFA25	Tinglongjian ('Between Hearing and Deafness')	Insertion: Indications:	Midway between Tingxue (OFA24) and SI19 (Tinggong). Vertical, 1-2 cun, with mouth open. Deafness.
OFA26	Tingling ('Hearing's Inspiration')	Insertion: Indications:	Midway between Tingxue (OFA24) and GB2 (Tinghui). Vertical, 1-2 cun, with mouth open. Tinnitus; deafness; deaf-mutism.
OFA27	Tingcong ('Hearing')	Insertion: Indications:	2 fen below GB2 (Tinghui). Vertical, 1½-2 cun. Deafness.
OFA28	Tingmin ('Hearing Sensitivity')	Insertion: Indications:	At lower root of ear-lobe. Vertical, 1½ cun. Deafness.
OFA29	Zhuding ('Pearl's Tip')	Insertion: Indications:	Tip of tragus of ear. Vertical, 3 fen. Diseases of ear; toothache.

Points in the Mouth

M1	Jinjin, Yuyue ('Gold Fluid, Jade Fluid')	Insertion: Indications:	On veins on both sides of frenulum of tongue. Bleed with prismatic needle. Aphasia with stiffness of tongue; continual vomiting; stomatitis; glossitis; tonsillitis.
M2	Haiquan ('Sea's Spring')	Insertion: Indications:	In the centre of the frenulum. Bleed. Spasm of diaphragm; glossitis; emaciation with thirst.
M3	Shezhu ('Tongue's Pillar')	Insertion: Indications:	At the intersection of the frenulum with the sublingual fold. Bleed. Heavy tongue; emaciation with thirst.
M4	Jianei ('Inside Cheek')	Insertion: Indications:	On the buccal mucosa in the mouth, level with the first molar. Slanted towards ear, ½-1 cun, or bleed. Facial paralysis; deafness; ulceration of mouth or gums.
M5	Juquan ('Gathering Spring')	Insertion: Indications:	In the centre of the tongue surface. Vertical, 2-3 fen. Paralysis of tongue; asthma.

Other Non-Meridial Points
HEAD AND NECK

OHN1	Waijinjin; Waiyuye ('Outer Gold Fluid; Outer Jade Fluid')	Insertion: Indications:	With head raised, 3 fen from mid-line and 1 cun above laryngeal prominence. Slanted to root of tongue, ½-1 cun. Stomatitis; aphasia from apoplexy; paralysis of tongue.
OHN2	Panglianquan (Beside Spring of Integrity')	Insertion: Indications:	½ cun lateral to CV23 (Lianquan). Vertical, ½-1 cun. Swollen tongue; disease of vocal cords.
OHN3	Hongyin ('Huge Sound')	Insertion: Indications:	½ cun beside laryngeal prominence. Vertical 3-5 fen. Acute and chronic laryngitis; disease of vocal cords.
OHN4	Zhiou ('Stop Vomiting')	Insertion: Indications:	Midway between CV22 (Tiantu) and CV23 (Lianquan). Sloped to CV22, ½-1 cun. Vomiting; excess phlegm.
OHN5	Qiying ('Cervical Lump of Qi')	Insertion: Indications:	Near St10 (Shuitu), on lateral superior side of swelling associated with goitre. Vertical, 1-1½ cun. Simple goitre; hyperthyroidism.
OHN6	Yaxue ('Mute Orifice')	Insertion: Indications:	A combination of four points, two on the front of the neck about 2 fen lateral to the mid-point between St9 (Renying) and St10 (Shuitu), and two on the back of the neck about 4 fen above GB20 (Fengchi). Vertical 1 cun. (Avoid carotid artery with the anterior points). Deaf-mutism; disease of vocal cords.
OHN7	Qiangyin ('Strong Sound')	Insertion: Indications:	2 cun lateral to laryngeal prominence, above and behind St9 (Renying). Towards root of tongue, ½-1 cun. Aphasia due to disease of vocal cords.
OHN8	Xiafutu ('Lower Support Prominence')	Insertion: Indications:	½ cun below Co18 (Futu). Slant upwards, 3 fen to 1½ cun. Goitre; tremor; paralysis of upper limb.
OHN9	Ronghou ('Behind Heaven's Contents')	Insertion: Indications:	1½ cun below TH17 (Yifeng), just posterior to SI17 (Tianrong). Vertical, ½-1 cun. Deafness; toothache; headache.

37

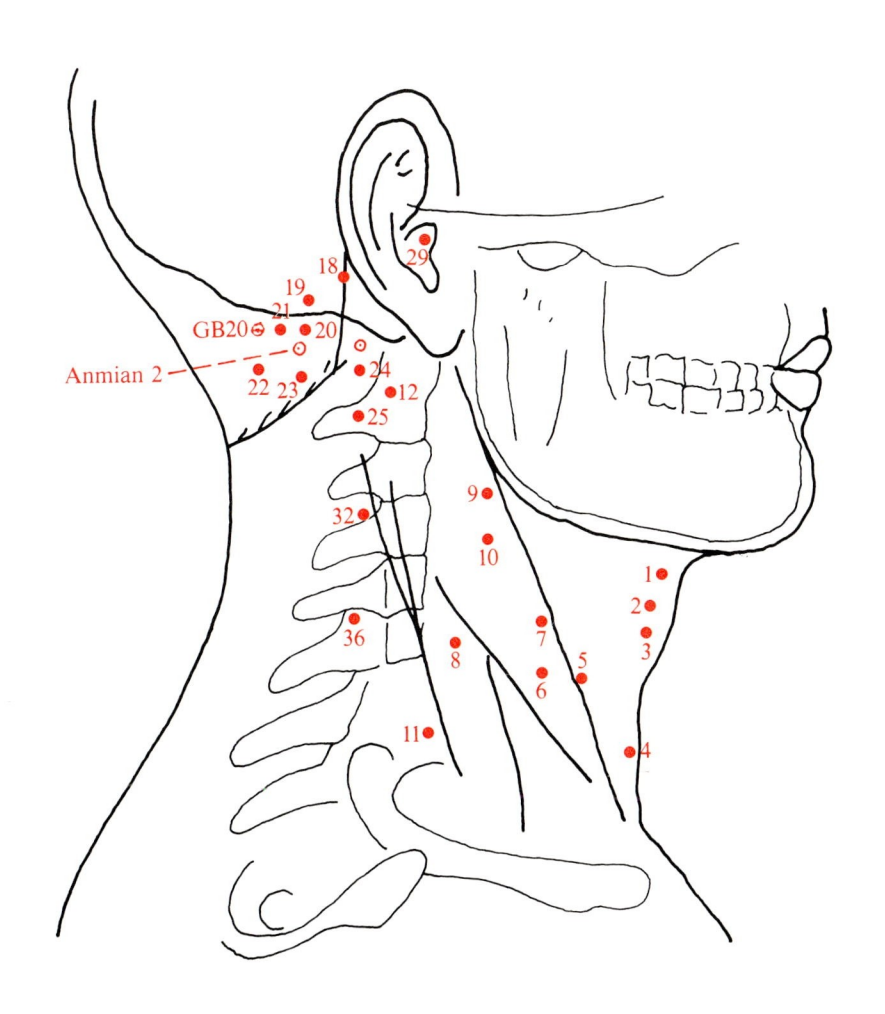

OHN10	Luojing ('Stiff Neck')		In middle of sternocleidomastoid muscle, below Ronghou (OHN9).
		Insertion:	Vertical, 1-1½ cun.
		Indications:	Stiff Neck.
OHN11	Huxi ('Breathing')		About 3 fen below the junction of the lateral margin of the sternocleidomastoid muscle with the jugular vein.
		Insertion:	Vertical, 5-8 fen.
		Indications:	Paralysis of respiratory muscles; diaphragmatic spasms; apnoea.
OHN12	Fengyan ('Wind's Cliff')		½ cun in front of the mid-point between the inferior border of the ear-lobe and GV15 (Yamen).
		Insertion:	Vertical, 1-1½ cun.
		Indications:	Insanity; hysteria; neurasthenia; neurotic headaches; sequelae of brain disease with mental retardation.
OHN13	Shangergen ('Upper Ear Root')		Middle of upper root of auricle.
		Insertion:	Slanted, ½-1 cun.
		Indications:	Hemiplegia; lateral sclerosis.
OHN14	Houcong ('Posterior Hearing')		Midway between upper auricular root and natural hairline at back of neck.
		Insertion:	Slanted, 3-5 fen.
		Indications:	Deafness.
OHN15	Houtinggong ('Posterior Palace of Hearing')		At auricular root, behind ear, level with SI19 (Tinggong).
		Insertion:	Slanted, ½-1 cun.
		Indications:	Deafness.
OHN16	Houtingxue ('Posterior Hearing Points')		Midway between SI19 (Tinggong) and Yilong (HN1).
		Insertion:	Slanted, ½-1 cun.
		Indications:	Deafness.
OHN17	Erbeijing-maisantiao ('Three Veins on Back of Ear')		On the three veins at the back of the auricle.
		Insertion:	Bleed.
		Indications:	Hordeolum; conjunctivitis; skin diseases.
OHN18	Yanchi ('Cliff's Pool')		At intersection of a line level with the highest point of the mastoid process and the natural hair-line.
		Insertion:	Vertical and slightly backwards, 1-1½ cun.
		Indications:	Glaucoma; vertigo; hypertension.
OHN19	Xingfen ('Excitement')		About ½ cun in a slanted direction above Anmian 2 (HN4), just posterior to the margin of the mastoid process.
		Insertion:	Vertical, ½-1 cun.
		Indications:	Bradycardia; idiocy after brain disease; hypersomnia.

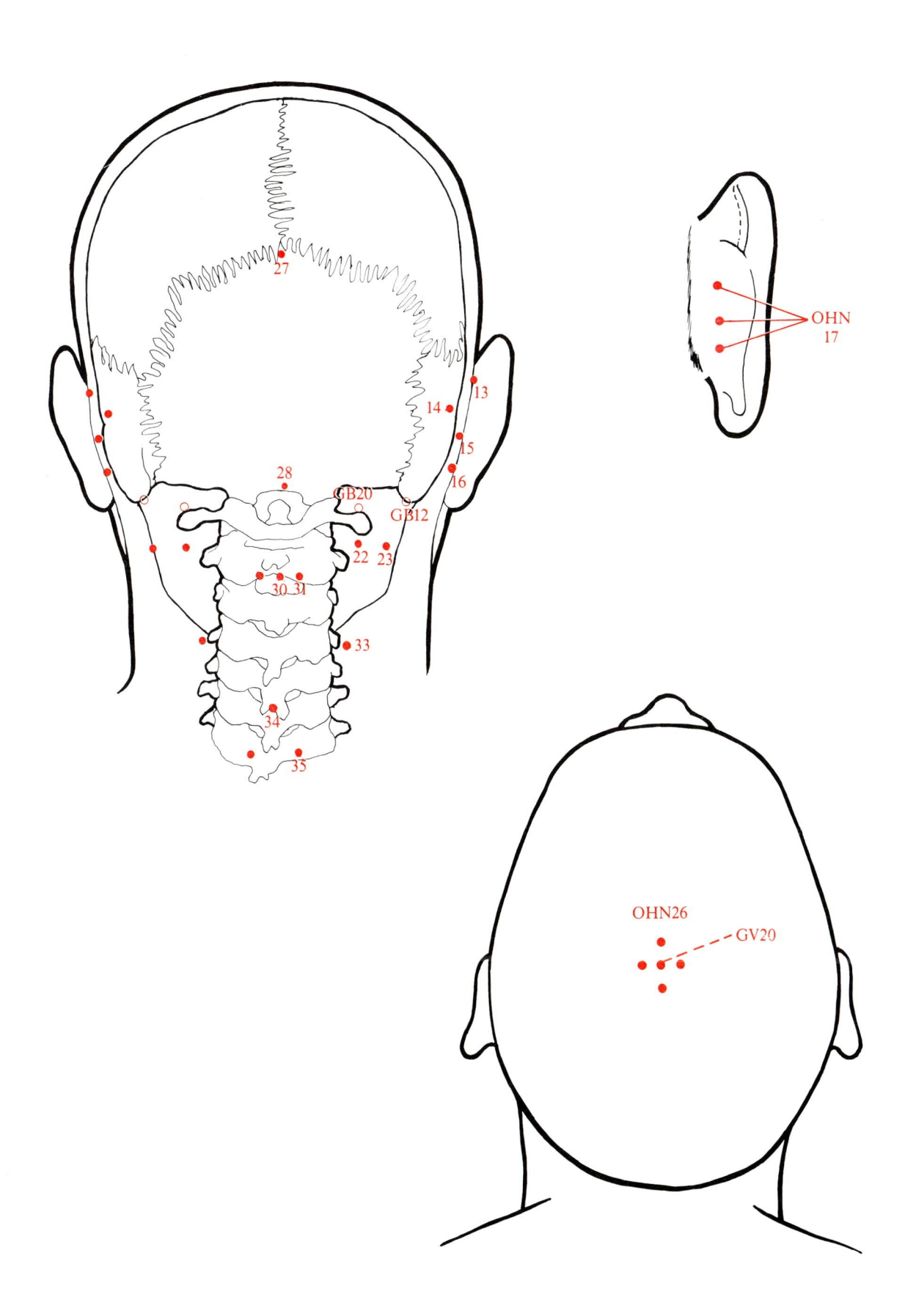

OHN20	Yaming ('Mute Call')	Insertion: Indications:	1 cun anterior to GB20 (Fengchi). Vertical, 1-1½ cun, to tip of nose. Deaf-mutism; pharyngolaryngitis.
OHN21	Chiqian ('Before the Pool')	Insertion: Indications:	½ cun anterior to GB20 (Fengchi). Slanted, 1-1½ cun, towards TH17 (Yifeng). Deafness; cataract.
OHN22	Chixia ('Below the Pool')	Insertion: Indications:	½ cun below GB20 (Fengchi). Vertical, 1-1½ cun. Occipital headache; glaucoma; retinitis pigmentosa.
OHN23	Tianting ('Heaven's Hearing')	Insertion: Indications:	½ cun below Anmian 2 (HN4). Vertical 1 cun. Deafness.
OHN24	Ximingxia ('Below Dim Light')	Insertion: Indications:	½ cun below Yiming (HN2). Vertical, 1½ cun. Deafness.
OHN25	Tongerdao ('Through the Ear Canal')	Insertion: Indications:	1 cun below Yiming (HN2). Slanted to ear-drum, 1-2 cun. Tinnitus; deafness.
OHN26	Sishencong ('Four Intelligence')	Insertion: Indications:	4 points, each 1 cun from GV20 (Baihui) anterior, posterior, and both sides. Slanted posteriorly, ½-1 cun. Headache and feeling of vertex fullness; vertigo; seizures; neurasthenia.
OHN27	Damen ('Big Door')	Insertion: Indications:	Median line of head, ½ cun posterior to GV18 (Qiangjian). Slanted posteriorly, ½ cun. Hemiplegia following stroke.
OHN28	Zhongjie ('Middle Connection')	Insertion: Indications:	7 fen above GV16 (Fengfu). Slanted to right or left, ½ cun. Hydrocephalus.
OHN29	Waierdaokou ('Opening of the External Ear Canal')	Insertion: Indications:	At the top of the auditory meatus. Vertical, 3-5 fen. Tinnitus; deafness.
OHN30	Xiayamen ('Lower Door of Muteness')	Insertion: Indications:	1 cun below GV15 (Yamen). Vertical, ½-1 cun. Sequelae of brain-disease.
OHN31	Fuyamen ('Secondary Door of Muteness')	Insertion: Indications:	½ cun lateral to Xiayamen (OHN30). Vertical, ½-1 cun. Sequelae of brain-disease.
OHN32	Jingzhong ('Middle of Neck')	Insertion: Indications:	2 cun below Anmian 2 (HN4), on the posterior border of the sternocleidomastoid muscle. Vertical or slanted upwards, ½-1 cun. Stiff and painful neck; hemiplegia.

OHN33	Xiaxinshi ('Lower New Recognition')	Insertion: Indications:	½ cun below Xinshi (HN8). Vertical, 1-1½ cun. Pituitary adenoma.
OHN34	Xinyi ('New One')	Insertion: Indications:	Between spinous processes of 5th and 6th cervicals. Slightly slanted, ½-1 cun. Incomplete maturation of cerebral cortex; seizures; psychosis.
OHN35	Dijia 1 ('Endemic Goitre')	Insertion: Indications:	One finger-width lateral and ½ cun above GV14 (Dazhui). Vertical, 1 cun. Endemic Goitre.
OHN36	Dijia 2 ('Endemic Goitre')	Insertion: Indications:	Level with the mid-point of the sternocleidomastoid muscle, 1 cun posteriorly. Vertical, ½ cun. Endemic Goitre.

Other Non-Meridial Points
CHEST AND ABDOMEN

OCA1	Xiaokuai ('Eliminate Lump')	Insertion: Indications:	At the top of the anterior axillary crease. Slant upwards, 1-1½ cun. Breast tumour.
OCA2	Chixue ('Red Orifice')	Insertion: Indications:	1 cun lateral to CV21 (Xuanji). Slanted upwards, ½-1 cun. (Downwards for intercostals). Cough; asthma; intercostal neuralgia.
OCA3	Xinleitou ('New Rib's Head')	Insertion: Indications:	2 points, beside the sternum in the first and second intercostal spaces. Slanted, 3-5 fen. Asthma; bronchitis; intercostal neuralgia; costal chondritis.
OCA4	Xiaoerjixiong ('Infantile Chicken Breast')	Insertion: Indications:	3 points, in the 2nd, 3rd and 4th intercostal spaces, abut 2½ cun from the mid-line. Moxa Pigeon-breast.
OCA5	Xiongdaji ('Pectoralis Major')	Insertion: Indications:	2 finger-widths lateral to the nipple. Slanted, 5-8 fen. Atrophy of pectoralis major muscle.
OCA6	Tanchuan ('Phlegm and Wheezing')	Insertion: Indications:	1¾ cun lateral to St16 (Yinchuang). Slanted, ½-1 cun. Chronic bronchitis; asthma.
OCA7	Longhan ('Dragon Jaw')	Insertion: Indications:	Midway between CV16 (Zhongting) and CV17 (Shanzhong). Slanted, ½-1 cun. Pain in the chest; stomach-ache.
OCA8	Zuoyi, Youyi ('Right and Left Propriety')	Insertion: Indications:	1 cun lateral and slightly superior to St18 (Rugen). Slanting, 3-5 fen. Mastitis; pleurisy; intercostal neuralgia.
OCA9	Ganshi ('Liver's Dwelling')	Insertion: Indications:	Directly below nipple, between 6th and 7th ribs. Slanted, 3-5 fen. Hepatomegaly; pain in liver area.
OCA10	Eni ('Hiccup')	Insertion: Indications:	Directly below nipple, in 7th intercostal space. Slanted, 3-5 fen, or moxa. Hiccups.
OCA11	Chuangxinmen ('Create New Door')	Insertion: Indications:	Just above 9th rib at its intercostal junction. Slanted, 5-8 fen. Chronic schistosomiasis.
OCA12	Shicang ('Granary')	Insertion: Indications:	3 cun lateral to CV12 (Zhongwan). Vertical, 1½-2 cun. Nephritis; peptic ulcer; indigestion; lack of appetite; menorrhagia.

43

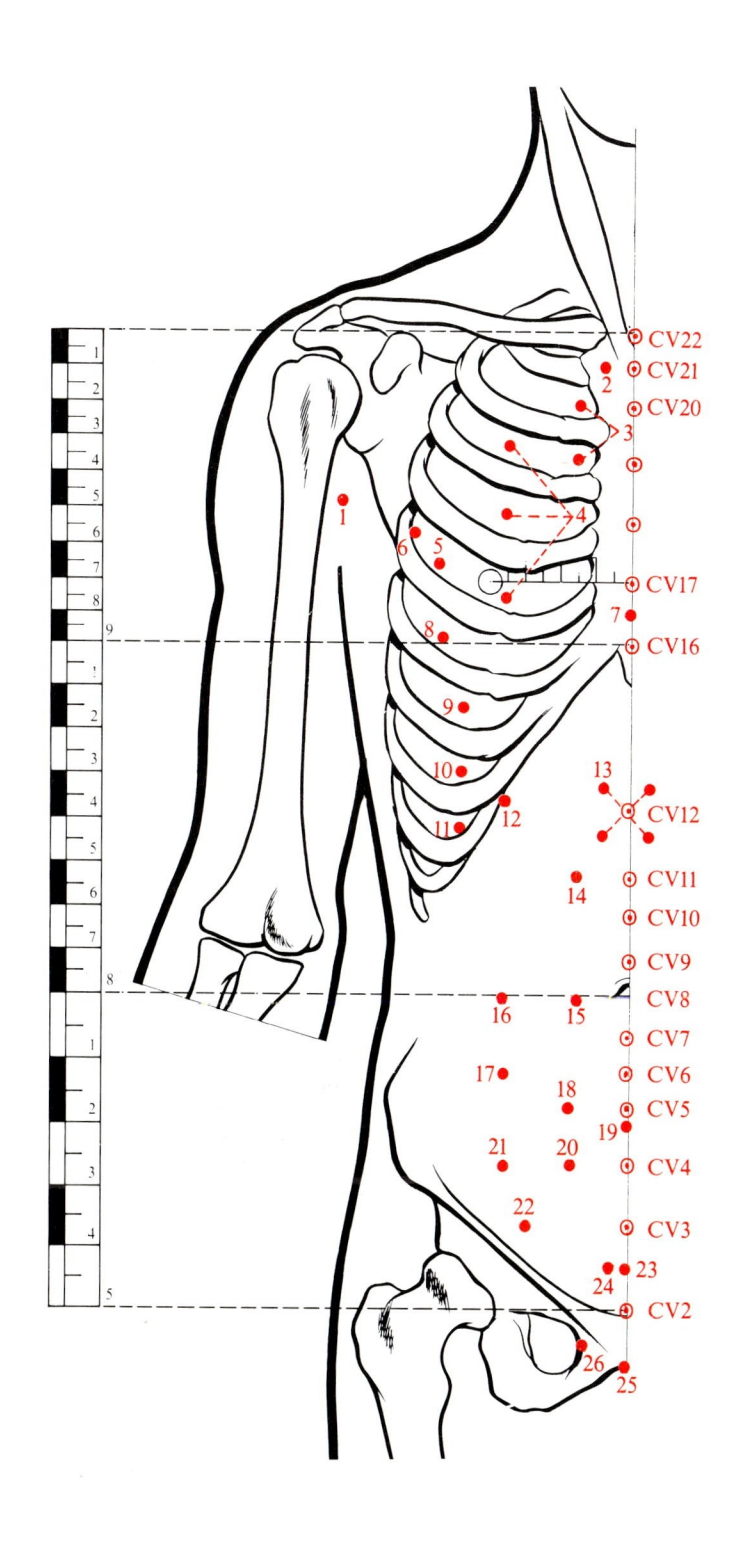

OCA13	Meihua ('Plum Blossom')		5 points, including CV12 (Zhongwan), the other four being, bilaterally, ½ cun above and below Ki19 (Yindu).
		Insertion:	Vertical, 1-1½ cun.
		Indications:	Indigestion; gastric ulcer; gastritis.
OCA14	Shiguan ('Food's Gate')		1 cun lateral to CV11 (Jianli).
		Insertion:	Vertical, 1½-2 cun.
		Indications:	Nephritis; indigestion; enteritis; belching.
OCA15	Hunshe ('Mingled Associations')		1 cun lateral to CV8 (Shenjue).
		Insertion:	Vertical, 1½-2 cun.
		Indications:	Dysentery; enteritis; indigestion.
OCA16	Tongbian ('Bowel Movement')		3 cun lateral to CV8 (Shenjue).
		Insertion:	Vertical, 1-2 cun.
		Indications:	Constipation due to paraplegia.
OCA17	Jingzhong ('Middle of Channel')		3 cun lateral to CV6 (Qihai).
		Insertion:	Vertical, 1½-2 cun.
		Indications:	Constipation; irregular menstruation; enteritis; peritonitis.
OCA18	Waisiman ('Outer Four Full')		1 cun lateral to Ki14 (Siman).
		Insertion:	Moxa.
		Indications:	Irregular menses.
OCA19	Jueyun ('Miscarriage')		3 fen below CV5 (Shimen).
		Insertion:	Moxa
		Indications:	Miscarriage; infantile diarrhoea.
OCA20	Yijing ('Spermatorr-hoea')		1 cun lateral to CV4 (Guanyuan).
		Insertion:	Vertical, 1½-2 cun.
		Indications:	Premature ejaculation; impotence; scrotal eczema.
OCA21	Qimen ('Qi's Door')		3 cun lateral to CV4 (Guanyuan).
		Insertion:	Vertical, 1½-2 cun.
		Indications:	Menorrhagia; sterility; orchitis; cystitis; puerperal leucorrhoea.
OCA22	Changyi ('Intestinal Remnant')		2½ cun lateral to CV3 (Zhongji).
		Insertion:	Vertical, 1-1½ cun.
		Indications:	Irregular menses; pain in penis; orchitis; adnexitis.
OCA23	Xiazhongji ('Below Middle Summit')		Midway between CV2 (Qugu) and CV3 (Zhongji).
		Insertion:	Slant to pubis, 2-2½ cun.
		Indications:	Incontinence due to paraplegia.
OCA24	Tingtou ('Erect Head')		½ cun below Ki12 (Dahe).
		Insertion:	Vertical, 1-1½ cun.
		Indications:	Prolapse of the uterus.
OCA25	Longmen ('Dragon's Gate')		On the midline of the inferior border of the pubic symphysis.
		Insertion:	Slanted ½-1 cun.
		Indications:	Abnormal uterine bleeding; incontinence; female infertility.

OCA26	Yinbian ('Beside Genitals')	Insertion: Indications:	On the lower border of the pubic symphysis, ½ cun lateral to the midline. Slant to midline, ½-1 cun. Incontinence or retention due to paraplegia.
OCA27	Qisbian ('Four Sides of Navel')		4 points, approximately 1 cun to the left and right, above and below the navel. 3 of these would be CV9 (Shuifen) and the bilateral Hunshe (OCA15) (Not illustrated).
		Insertion: Indications:	Vertical, 1-1½ cun, or moxa. Acute gastro-enteritis; spastic stomach; indigestion; oedema.

Other Non-Meridial Points
DORSAL AND LUMBAR

ODL1 1a, b & c	Jisanxue ('Three Vertebral Orifices')	Insertion: Indications:	1 cun below and ½ cun lateral to GV15 (Yamen); ½ cun lateral to D2 and ½ cun lateral to L2 vertebrae. Slanted, ½-1 cun, or moxa. Spondylitis; myelitis; disorders of spine and cord; neuralgia of back.
ODL2	Zhinao, Nos.1-5 ('Heal Brain')	Insertion: Indications:	5 points on the midline between the spinous processes of C2/3/4/5/6/7. Vertical 1-1½ cun. (Withdraw immediately if strong sensation felt). Diseases of the brain.
ODL3	Liujing-zhuipang ('Beside the 6th Cervical Vertebra')	Insertion: Indications:	½ cun lateral to spinous process of C6. Vertical, ½-1 cun. Rhinitis; loss of sense of smell.
ODL4	Chonggu ('Lofty Bone')	Insertion: Indications:	Below spinous process of C6. (This is the 5th of the Zhinao (ODL2) points.) Slanting, ½-1 cun. Asthma; common cold; bronchitis; stiff neck; epilepsy.
ODL5	Qijingzhuipang ('Beside 7th Cervical Vertebra')	Insertion: Indications:	½ cun lateral to spinous process of C7. Vertical, ½-1 cun. Tonsillitis; pharyngitis.
ODL6	Waidingchuan ('Outer Stop Wheezing')	Insertion: Indications:	1½ cun lateral to GV14 (Dazhui). Slanted towards spine, ½-¾ cun. Bronchitis; asthma.
ODL7	Baizhongfeng ('Hundred Kinds of Wind')	Insertion: Indications:	2.3 cun lateral to GV14 (Dazhui). Slanted, ½-1 cun. Pain at the back of the shoulder; urticaria; apoplexy.
ODL8	Jiehexue ('Tuberculosis Orifice')	Insertion: Indications:	3½ cun lateral to GV14 (Dazhui). Vertical, ½-¾ cun. Tuberculosis.
ODL9	Chuchueh ('Resist Pain')	Insertion: Indications:	Slightly below medial side of upper border of scapula. Slanted, ½-1 cun. Pain in scapula; hysteria.
ODL10	Jugoxia ('Below Great Bone')	Insertion: Indications:	2 cun below Co16 (Jugu). Vertical, 1-2 cun. Diseases of the shoulder joint and tissues.

ODL11	Feirexue ('Lung Heat Orifice')	Insertion: Indications:	½ cun lateral to spinous process of D3 (Jiaji point). Slanted to spine, ½-1 cun. Bronchitis; pleurisy; pneumonia; pain in back.
ODL12	Juqueshu ('Great Palace Hollow')	Insertion: Indications:	Below tip of spinous process of D4. Slanting, ½-1 cun. Bronchitis; asthma, heart trouble; intercostal neuralgia.
ODL13	Weirexue ('Stomach Heat Orifice')	Insertion: Indications:	½ cun lateral to spinous process of D4 (Jiaji point). Slanted to spine, ½-1 cun. Vomiting; swollen and painful gums; stomach-ache.
ODL14	Ganrexue ('Liver Heat Orifice')	Insertion: Indications:	½ cun lateral to spinous process of D5 (Jiaji point). Slanted to spine, ½-1 cun. Bronchitis; hepatitis; cholecystitis; intercostal neuralgia.
ODL15	Huanmen ('Affliction's Door')	Insertion: Indications:	Slightly above Bl15 (Xinshu). Moxa. Bronchitis; asthma; T.B. of lung; general debility after long illness.
ODL16	Pirexue ('Spleen Heat Orifice')	Insertion: Indications:	½ cun lateral to spinous process of D6 (Jiaji point). Slanted to spine, ½-1 cun. Hepatitis; pancreatitis; splenomegaly.
ODL17	Shenrexue ('Kidney Heat Orifice')	Insertion: Indications:	½ cun lateral to spinous process of D7 (Jiaji point). Slanted to spine, ½-1 cun. Nephritis; infection of genito-urinary tract.
ODL18	Qichuan ('Wheezing')	Insertion: Indications:	2 cun lateral to spinous process of D7, slightly above Bl17 (Geshu). Slanted to spine, ½-1 cun. Bronchitis; asthma; pleurisy.
ODL19	Anmian 3 ('Peaceful Sleep')	Insertion: Indications:	½ cun lateral to Bl17 (Geshu). Slanted, ½-1 cun. Insomnia; irritability.
ODL20	Yinkou ('Silver Mouth')	Insertion: Indications:	At the inferior angle of the scapula. Slanted, ½-1 cun. Haemoptysis; intercostal neuralgia; pneumonia.
ODL21	Yishu ('Pancreas Hollow')	Insertion: Indications:	1½ cun lateral to spinous process of D8. Slanted to spine, ½-1 cun. Diabetes; gastric disorders; intercostal neuralgia.
ODL22	Bazhuixia ('Below Eighth Vertebra')	Insertion: Indications:	Below spinous process of D8. Slanted slightly upwards, ½-1 cun. Diabetes; hepatitis; intercostal neuralgia; malaria.

ODL23	Weiguanxiashu ('Stomach's Lower Hinge Hollow')	Insertion: Indications:	1½ cun lateral to the lower border of the spinous process of D8. Oblique 5-7 fen, or moxa. Vomiting; abdominal pain.
ODL24	Jianming 5 ('Strengthens Brightness')	Insertion: Indications:	1½ cun lateral to spinous process of D9, about ½ cun above Bl18 (Ganshu). Vertical, 5-8 fen. Optic atrophy; retinitis.
ODL25	Shubian ('Beside the Axis')	Insertion: Indications:	1 cun lateral to the spinous process of D10. Slanted to spine, ½-1 cun. Gastric disorders; disorders of liver and gall-bladder.
ODL26	Zhuoyu ('Bathing the Unclean')	Insertion: Indications:	2½ cun lateral to the spinous process of D10. Slanted to spine, ½-1 cun. Diseases of liver and gall-bladder; anorexia.
ODL27	Dianxian ('Epilepsy')	Insertion: Indications:	Midway between GV14 (Dazhui) and the tip of the coccyx — usually on the spinous process of D11. Moxa. Epilepsy and convulsions.
ODL28	Jiegu ('Connecting Bone')	Insertion: Indications:	In depression below spinous process of D12. Slanted slightly upwards, ½-1 cun. Anal prolapse; indigestion; gastralgia; enteritis.
ODL29	Zhongjiaoshu ('Middle Burner's Hollow')	Insertion: Indications:	2 cun lateral to D12 vertebra. Slanted 75° slightly upwards. On left side 1½-2 cun, on right side superficial only. Chronic schistosomiasis.
ODL30	Kuiyangxue ('Ulcer Orifice')	Insertion: Indications:	2 cun lateral to Bl45 (Weicang). Slanted 5-8 fen. Gastric and duodenal ulcers.
ODL31	Pigen ('Lump's Root')	Insertion: Indications:	3½ cun lateral to lower end of spinous process of L1. Vertical, 1-1½ cun. Hepatomegaly; splenomegaly; nephritis; enteritis; lumbago.
ODL32	Xuechou ('Blood Worry')	Insertion: Indications:	Above spinous process of L2. Vertical, 1-1½ cun. Haemorrhagic disorders.
ODL33	Changfeng ('Intestinal Wind')	Insertion: Indications:	1 cun lateral to lower end of spinous process of L2. Vertical, 1-1½ cun. Haemorrhoids; stomach and intestinal disorders; nocturia.
ODL34	Xuefu ('Blood's Residence')	Insertion: Indications:	4 cun lateral to the spinous process of L2. Vertical, 1-1½ cun. Amenorrhoea; ovarian hyperplasia; hepatomegaly; splenomegaly; spermatorrhoea.

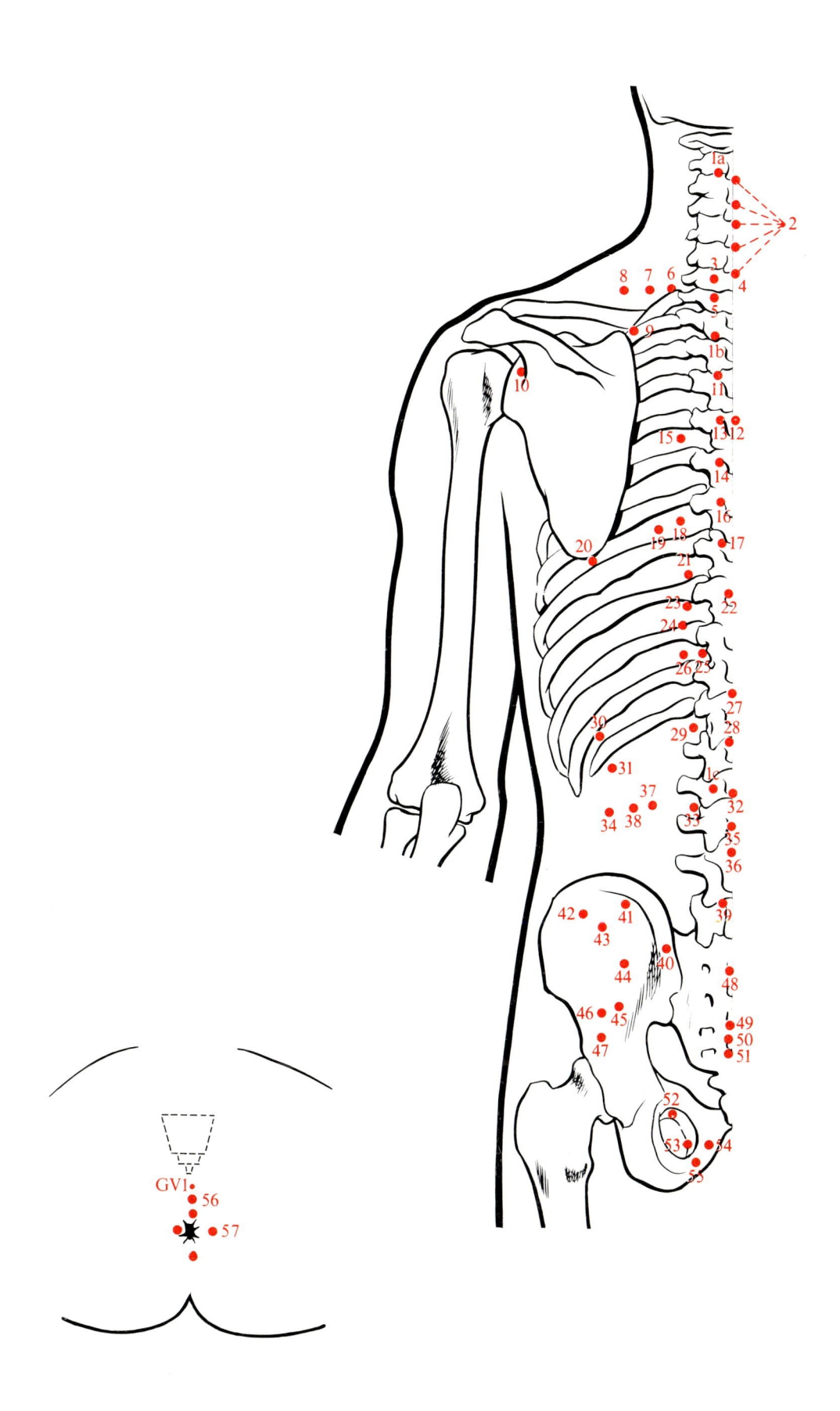

ODL35	Zhuzhang ('Bamboo Cane')	Insertion: Indications:	Above spinous process of L3. Moxa. Haemorrhoids; anal prolapse; enteritis; intestinal T.B.; blood in stool.
ODL36	Xiajishu ('Lower Level Hollow')	Insertion: Indications:	Below spinous process of L3. Slanted slightly upwards, 1-1½ cun. Low-back pain; cystitis; paralysis of lower limb.
ODL37	Shenxin ('Kidney New')	Insertion: Indications:	3-5 fen lateral to Bl23 (Shenshu). Slanted 45° towards spine, 1-1½ cun. Rheumatic heart disease.
ODL38	Zhantan ('Fight Paralysis')	Insertion: Indications:	2½ cun lateral to the spinous process of L2. Slanted, 2-3 cun. Paraplegia.
ODL39	Xishang ('Above the Creek')	Insertion: Indications:	3-5 fen lateral to the interspinal process between L4 and L5 (Jiaji point). Slant to mid-line, ½-1 cun. Chronic pain in low-back and leg.
ODL40	Qiahoushangji ('Posterior Superior Iliac Spine')	Insertion: Indications:	At the posterior superior iliac spine. Vertical, 1-2 cun. Paralysis of lower limb.
ODL41	Yaoyi ('Lower Back Propriety')	Insertion: Indications:	3 cun lateral to spinous process of L4. Vertical, 1-2 cun. Lumbago; menorrhagia.
ODL42	Tiaoyue ('Leap')	Insertion: Indications:	2 cun below the highest point of the iliac crest. Vertical, 2-3 cun. Sequelae of poliomyelitis.
ODL43	Zhongkong ('Middle Space')	Insertion: Indications:	3½ cun lateral to spinous process of L5. Vertical, 1½-2 cun. Lumbago.
ODL44	Yaogan ('Lower Back's Root')	Insertion: Indications:	3 cun lateral to spinous process of S1. Vertical 2-3 cun. Sacro-iliac joint disorders; disorders of lower limbs.
ODL45	Maigen ('Vessel's Root')	Insertion: Indications:	3 cun lateral and ½ cun inferior to second sacral foramen. Vertical, 3-5 cun. Buerger's disease.
ODL46	Huanyue ('Encircling')	Insertion: Indications:	The point at which a line drawn from the great trochanter to the spinous process of L5 crosses one drawn from the anterior superior iliac spine to the coccyx. Vertical, 2-2½ cun. Paralysis of lower limb.

ODL47	Tunzhong ('Middle of Buttock')	Insertion: Indications:	At the apex of an imaginary equilateral triangle the base of which is a line drawn between the great trochanter and the ischial tuberosity. Vertical, 2-3 cun. Sciatica; paralysis of the lower limb; urticaria; cold feet.
ODL48	Jiuqi ('Wild Pigeon Willow')	Insertion: Indications:	Below spinous process of S1. Moxa. Abnormal uterine bleeding; leucorrhagia.
ODL49	Xiazhui ('Lower Vertebra')	Insertion: Indications:	Below spinous process of S3. Slanted, ½-1 cun. Irregular menses; enteritis; gonococcal urethritis.
ODL50	Yutian ('Jade Field')	Insertion: Indications:	Below spinous process of S4. Slanted, ½-1 cun, or moxa. Low-back pain; spasm of gastrocnemius muscle; difficult labour.
ODL51	Pinxueling ('Anaemic's Inspiration')	Insertion: Indications:	Above spinous process of S5, 3 fen below ODL50. Moxa. Anaemia.
ODL52	Dayan ('Strike Eye')	Insertion: Indications:	2½ cun lateral and ½ cun below GV2 (Yaoshu). Vertical, 2-3 cun. Incontinence of faeces and urine due to paraplegia.
ODL53	Bikong ('Close Hole')	Insertion: Indications:	2 cun lateral to the tip of the coccyx. Vertical, 3-4 cun. Sciatica; paralysis of lower limb.
ODL54	Libian ('Regulate Excretion')	Insertion: Indications:	1 cun lateral to the tip of the coccyx. Vertical, 1½-2 cun. Incontinence of faeces and urine due to paraplegia.
ODL55	Pangqiang ('Beside Strength')	Insertion: Indications:	1½ cun lateral to GV1 (Changqiang). Slanted upwards, 3-4 cun. Prolapse of anus or uterus.
ODL56	Xiajiaoshu ('Lower Burner's Hollow')	Insertion: Indications:	Midway between GV1 (Changqiang) and the anus. Slanted upwards, 1½-2 cun. Chronic schistosomiasis. Can stimulate the nerves of the pelvic plexus.
ODL57	Gangmensixue ('Four Anal Orifices')	Insertion: Indications:	Four points in all, at ½ cun above, below and on each side of the anus. Vertical, 1-2 cun. Incontinence of urine and faeces due to paraplegia.
ODL58	Jifeng ('Vertebral Seams')	Insertion: Indications:	A series of points 4½ cun lateral to the interspinous spaces from D1 to L5. Slanted 3-5 fen. (Not too deep). Spondylitis; myelitis.

ODL59	Liuhua, Bahua ('Six Flowers, Eight Flowers')		Eight points in all, on either side of the spine. The first two are the base angles of an equilateral triangle with sides 2 cun long and its apex at GV14. The mid-point of the base line forms the apex of a second triangle, with the next two points at the extremities of its base-line. This process is repeated down the spine for a series of four triangles, giving the eight points.
		Insertion:	Slanted, ½-1 cun towards spine. In chronic conditions, moxa.
		Indications:	Bronchitis; asthma; anaemia; T.B. of lung; general debility after long illness.

Other Non-Meridial Points
ARM AND HAND
(anterior aspect)

OAR1	Tianling ('Heaven's Spirit')	Insertion: Indications:	1 cun above and ½ cun medial to the apex of the anterior axillary crease. Slanted laterally, 1-2 cun. Pain in the shoulder; mental illness.
OAR2	Yeling ('Axilla's Spirit')	Insertion: Indications:	½ cun above the anterior axillary crease. Vertical, 1-2 cun. Pain in the shoulder; mental illness.
OAR3	Zhitan 1 ('Head Paralysis')	Insertion: Indications:	In the hollow below the acromial end of the clavicle. Vertical, 1-2 cun. Diseases of the shoulder joint and soft tissues; hemiplegia due to stroke.
OAR4	Xiaxiabai ('Lower Gallantry')	Insertion: Indications:	3 cun distal to Lu4 (Xiabai). Vertical, 1-1½ cun. Palpitations; rheumatic heart disease.
OAR5	Zequian ('Before the Marsh')	Insertion: Indications:	1 cun distal and slightly medial to Lu5 (Chize), on a straight line from the middle finger. Vertical, 1 cun. Paralysis of upper limb; goitre.
OAR6	Zexia ('Below the Marsh')	Insertion: Indications:	2 cun distal to Lu5 (Chize). Vertical, 1 cun. Toothache; pain in forearm; haemorrhoids.
OAR7	Xishang ('Above Xi')	Insertion: Indications:	3 cun proximal to HC4 (Ximen). Vertical, 1 cun. Palpitations; valvular disease of heart; mastitis.
OAR8	Dingshu ('Carbuncle's Hollow')	Insertion: Indications:	4 cun proximal to the ulnar end of the wrist crease. Moxa. Carbuncle.
OAR9	Shoujinmen ('Hand's Golden Door')	Insertion: Indications:	3½ cun proximal to the middle of the wrist crease. Vertical, ½-1 cun. Scrofula.
OAR10	Neiyangchi ('Inner Yang's Pool')	Insertion: Indications:	1 cun distal to middle of wrist crease. Vertical, 3-5 fen. 'Swan-palm' paralysis; stomatitis; infantile convulsions; pain in larynx and pharynx.
OAR11	Xiaotianxin ('Little Heaven's Heart')	Insertion: Indications:	1½ cun distal to the middle of the wrist crease. Vertical, 3-5 fen. Rheumatic heart disease; palpitations.

OAR12	Banmen ('Board's Door')	Insertion: Indications:	1 cun internal to Lu10 (Yuji), medial to thenar eminence. Vertical, 3-5 fen. Asthma; tonsillitis.
OAR13	Neihegu ('Inner Adjoining Valleys')	Insertion: Indications:	Slightly lateral and proximal to the head of the second metacarpal. Slanted to Co4 (Hegu), 1-1½ cun. Stiff neck.
OAR14	Panglaogong ('Beside Labour's Palace')	Insertion: Indications:	About one finger-width to the ulnar side of HC8 (Laogong). Vertical, 3-5 fen. Tonsillitis; numbness of fingers; toothache.
OAR15	Yatong ('Toothache')	Insertion: Indications:	1 cun below the metacarpophalangeal crease, between 3rd and 4th metacarpal bones. Vertical, ½ cun. Toothache.
OAR16	Shouzhongping ('Mid-Hand Level')	Insertion: Indications:	In the middle of the transverse crease of the metacarpophalangeal joint of the middle finger. Vertical, 2-3 fen. Stomatitis.
OAR17	Zhizhang ('Finger Palm')	Insertion: Indications:	Between the metacarpophalangeal joints of the middle and 3rd fingers, closer to the middle finger. Vertical, ½-1 cun. Insomnia; loss of memory; psychosis; seizures.
OAR18	Fengyan ('Wind's Ear')	Insertion: Indications:	At the radial end of the transverse crease of the interphalangeal joint of the thumb. Prick only. Night blindness.
OAR19	Muzhijie-hengwen ('Transverse Crease of Thumb Joint')	Insertion: Indications:	In the middle of the interphalangeal crease of the thumb. Moxa. Corneal nebula or pannus.

55

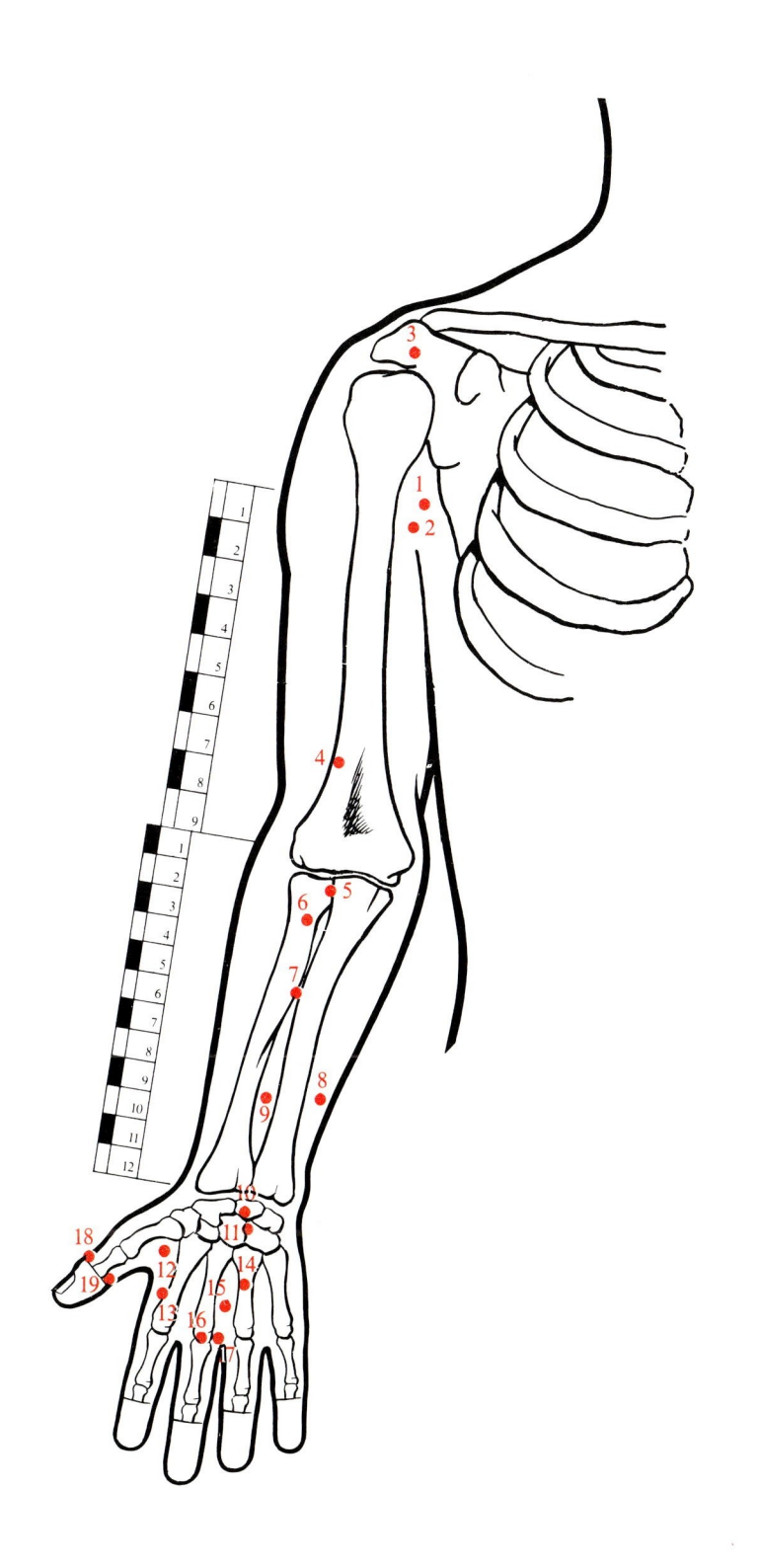

Other Non-Meridial Points
ARM AND HAND
(posterior aspect)

OAR20	Jianming ('See Brightness')	Insertion: Indications:	½ cun posterior to the 'Deltoid V' on the upper arm. Slanted upwards, 1-2 cun. Diseases of the eye; paralysis and paresis of the upper limb.
OAR21	Shenzhou ('Extend Elbow')	Insertion: Indications:	3 finger-widths above the olecranon, on the ulnar aspect. Vertical, 1-1½ cun. Stiffness of the elbow joint (particularly after fracture of the arm).
OAR22	Zhiyang ('Stop Itching')	Insertion: Indications:	1 cun above Co12 (Zhouliao). Slanted towards shoulder, 2 cun. Urticaria; allergic dermatitis; pruritis.
OAR23	Shangquchi ('Upper Crooked Pool')	Insertion: Indications:	1½ cun above Co11 (Quchi). Vertical, 1-2 cun. Paralysis of upper arm.
OAR24	Xinquchi ('New Crooked Pool')	Insertion: Indications:	½ cun above Co11 (Quchi). Vertical, 1-2 cun. Hypertension.
OAR25	Sanchi ('Three Pools')	Insertion: Indications:	Three points:- Co11 (Quchi), and two points at 1 cun above and 1 cun below it. Vertical, 1-1½ cun. Pain in elbow and arm; sinusitis.
OAR26	Zhoujian ('Elbow's tip')	Insertion: Indications:	At the tip of the olecranon when the elbow is flexed. Moxa. Scrofula; abscessed carbuncle.
OAR27	Zhoushu ('Elbow's Hollow')	Insertion: Indications:	At the back of the elbow, between the olecranon and the lateral epicondyle, when the elbow is flexed. Vertical, 3 fen. Pain in elbow joint.
OAR28	Sanliwai ('Three Outside Measures')	Insertion: Indications:	On forearm, 2 cun below and one finger-width lateral to Co11 (Quchi). Vertical, 1-2 cun. Paralysis of arm; sprain.
OAR29	Yingxia ('Below the Olecranon')	Insertion: Indications:	3 cun below the olecranon, between the radius and the ulna. Vertical, 1-2 cun. Paralysis of arm; deafness.

OAR30	Niushangxue ('Sprain's Orifice')	Insertion: Indications:	¼ of the distance from Co11 (Quchi) to TH4 (Yangchi). Very slightly medial to Co9 (Shanglian). Vertical, 1-2 cun. Acute low-back sprain.
OAR31	Chirao ('Ulna and Radius')	Insertion: Indications:	6 cun proximal to the middle of the dorsal wrist crease. Vertically through to the other side of the arm, without piercing the skin on the anterior aspect. Paralysis of arm; mental illness.
OAR32	Luoshang ('Above Connection')	Insertion: Indications:	3 cun proximal to TH5 (Waiguan). Vertical, 1-2 cun. Paralysis of arm; deafness.
OAR33	Xiawenliu ('Lower Warm Slide')	Insertion: Indications:	2 cun proximal to the radial end of the dorsal wrist crease. Vertical, 3-5 fen. Toothache of lower jaw.
OAR34	Cunping ('Unit Level')	Insertion: Indications:	1 cun proximal and 4 fen radially from the middle of the dorsal wrist crease. Vertical, ½-1 cun. Shock; heart failure.
OAR35	Zhongquan ('Middle Spring')	Insertion: Indications:	In the depression on the dorsum of the wrist between Co5 (Yangxi) and TH4 (Yangchi). Vertical, 3-5 fen. Asthma, bronchitis; corneal opacity; gastralgia; arthritis of wrist joint.
OAR36	Yaotang 1, 2 and 3 ('Low Back Pain')	Insertion: Indications:	Three points on the dorsum of the hand, between the bases of the 2nd and 3rd, 3rd and 4th, and 4th and 5th metacarpal bones. Slanted towards the wrist, 1-1½ cun. Yaotang 1 — Pain from injury to head, low-back and lower limbs. Yaotang 2 — Pain from injury to chest or limbs. Yaotang 3 — Pain from injury to lower back and limbs.
OAR37	Shanghouxi ('Upper Back Creek')	Insertion: Indications:	Between SI3 (Houxi) and SI4 (Wangu). Vertical, ½-1 cun. Deaf-mutism; numbness of fingers.
OAR38	Tongling ('Painful Spirit')	Insertion: Indications:	1 cun proximal to the knuckles between the 3rd and 4th metacarpal bones. Slanted to wrist, 1-1½ cun. Headache; toothache; stomach-ache.
OAR39	Luolingwu ('Stiff-neck One Half')	Insertion: Indications:	½ cun proximal to Luozhen (AR14). Slanted, ½-1 cun. Stiff neck; hypertension; stomach cramps.
OAR40	Hubian ('Beside the Tiger')	Insertion: Indications:	Between Co3 (Sanjian) and Co4 (Hegu). Slanted to SI3 (Houxi), 1-2 cun. Hysteria; psychosis; convulsions.

58

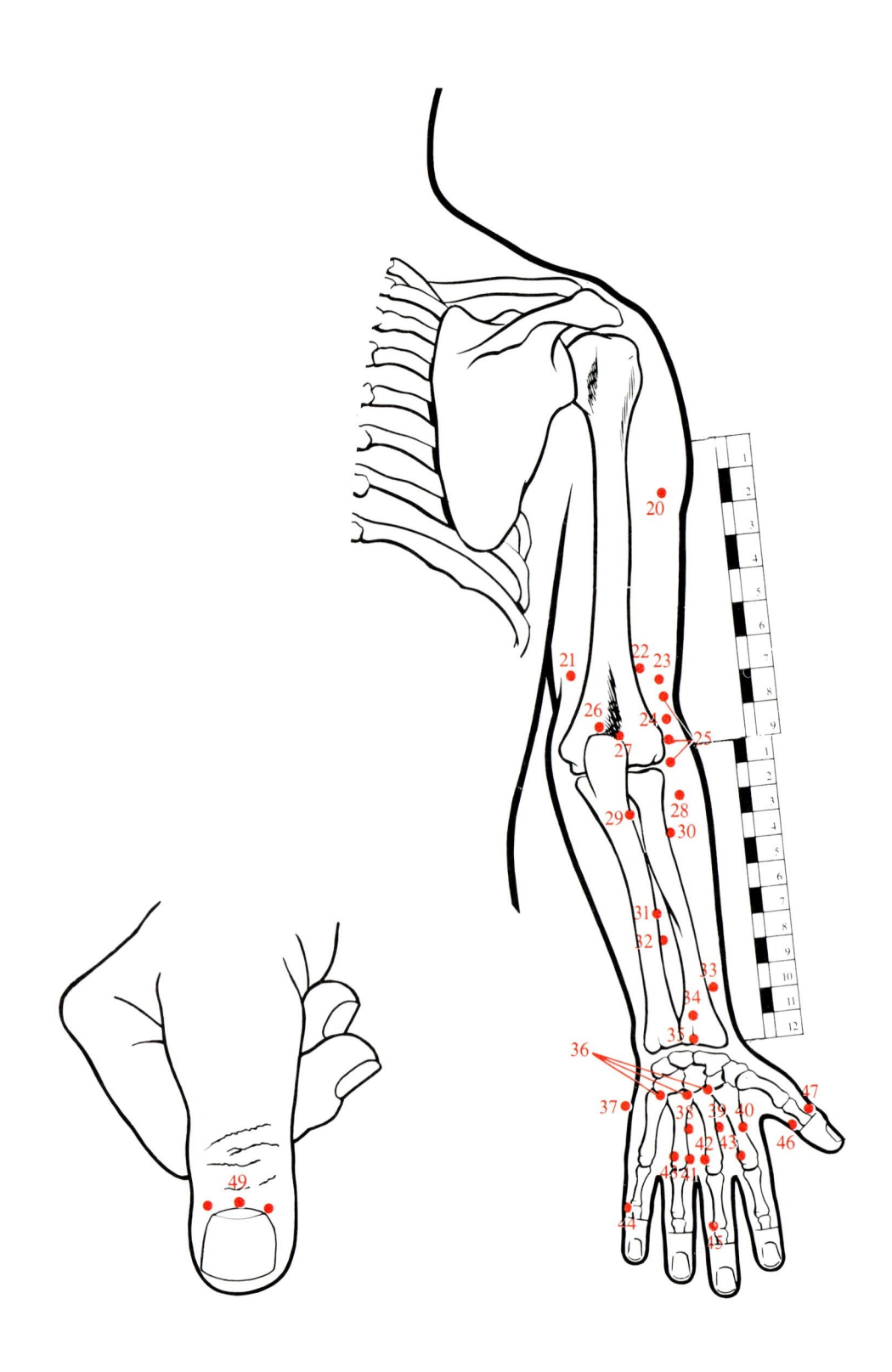

OAR41	Nuemen ('Malaria's Door')	Insertion: Indications:	On the dorsum between the knuckles of the 3rd and 4th metacarpal bones. Slanted, ½-1 cun. Malaria; ophthalmic disorders; scabies.
OAR42	Quanjian ('Fist's Tip')	Insertion: Indications:	On the knuckle of the middle finger. Bleed or moxa. Ophthalmic disorders; sore throat.
OAR43	Wuhu ('Five Tigers')	Insertion: Indications:	Two points, on the knuckles of the index and 3rd fingers. Insert with fist clenched, slanted 2-3 fen, or moxa. Stiff neck; sciatica; spasm of fingers.
OAR44	Xiaogukong ('Little Bone's Space')	Insertion: Indications:	In the middle of the proximal interphalangeal joint of the little finger. Moxa. Ophthalmic disorders; sore throat; arthritis of fingers.
OAR45	Zhongkui ('Middle Eminence')	Insertion: Indications:	In the middle of the proximal interphalangeal joint of the middle finger. Moxa. Vomiting; hiccups; oesophageal spasm; epistaxis.
OAR46	Mingyan ('Bright Eyes')	Insertion: Indications:	At the ulnar end of the palmar interphalangeal crease of the thumb. Prick. Conjunctivitis; night blindness; tonsillitis; infantile gastro-intestinal disorders.
OAR47	Dagukong ('Big Bone's Space')	Insertion: Indications:	Middle of the dorsal aspect of the interphalangeal joint of the thumb. Moxa. Ophthalmic disorders; vomiting and diarrhoea.
OAR48	Shiwang ('Ten Kings')	Insertion: Indications:	Ten points, in the centre of each finger-tip (just below the Shixuan (AR16) points). Prick. Acute gastro-enteritis; heat exhaustion; common cold.
OAR49	Sanshang ('Three Merchants')	Insertion: Indications:	Three points in line at the base of the thumb-nail. Prick. Influenza; tonsillitis; fever; parototis.

Other Non-Meridial Points
LEG AND FOOT

OLE1	Jiankua ('Strengthen Thigh')	Insertion: Indications:	(Lateral) Midway between the crest of the ilium and the greater trochanter. Vertical, 2-3 cun. Hemiplegia; paraplegia.
OLE2	Kuanjiu ('Acetabulum')	Insertion: Indications:	(Lateral) ½ cun directly above the trochanter. Vertical, 1½-2 cun. 'Relaxed' hip-joint from poliomyelitis.
OLE3	Qiangkua ('Strong Thigh')	Insertion: Indications:	(Lateral) 2 cun below the greater trochanter, at the posterior border of the femur. Vertical, 2½-3½ cun. Paraplegia.
OLE4	Xinhuantiao ('New Encircling Leap')	Insertion: Indications:	(Posterior) 3 cun lateral to coccyx. Vertical, 3-4 cun. Sciatica; paralysis of leg.
OLE5	Yinkang ('Yin's Excess')	Insertion: Indications:	(Posterior) 1½ cun medial to Bl50 (Chengfu). Vertical, 1-3 cun. Sciatica; sequelae of poliomyelitis.
OLE6	Yangkang ('Yang's Excess')	Insertion: Indications:	(Posterior) 1½ cun lateral to Bl50 (Chengfu). Vertical, 1-3 cun. Sciatica; sequelae of poliomyelitis.
OLE7	Jiaoling ('Straightening's Inspiration)	Insertion: Indications:	(Anterior) 3 cun below Li10 (Wuli). Vertical, 1-3 cun. Hemiplegia; sequelae of poliomyelitis; cholecystitis.
OLE8	Qiabinzhong ('Between Ilium and Knee')	Insertion: Indications:	(Anterior) 3 cun above and 1 cun lateral to St32 (Futu). Vertical, 1-2 cun. Arthritis of knee; paralysis of leg; low-back pain.
OLE9	Guantu ('Hinge and Rabbit')	Insertion: Indications:	(Anterior) Midway between St31 (Biguan) and St32 (Futu). Vertical, 1-2 cun. Enteritis; stomach-ache; sequelae of poliomyelitis.
OLE10	Yinshang ('Above the Abundance')	Insertion: Indications:	(Posterior) 2 cun above Bl51 (Yinmen). Vertical, 1-2 cun. Sciatica; sequelae of poliomyelitis.
OLE11	Qianjin ('Advance')	Insertion: Indications:	(Lateral) 2½ cun above GB31 (Fengshi). Vertical, 1½-2½ cun. Hemiplegia; paraplegia; sequelae of poliomyelitis.
OLE12	Shangfengshi ('Upper Market of Wind')	Insertion: Indications:	(Lateral) 2 cun above GB31 (Fengshi). Vertical, 1-2 cun. Sciatica; hemiplegia; sequelae of poliomyelitis.

OLE13	Xinfutu ('New Hidden Rabbit')	Insertion: Indications:	(Anterior) 3 fen lateral to St32 (Futu). Vertical, 1-2 cun. Arthritis of knee; paralysis of lower limb.
OLE14	Shenxi ('Kidney's Connection')	Insertion: Indications:	(Anterior) 1 cun below St32 (Futu). Vertical, 1-1½ cun. Diabetes; paralysis of lower limb.
OLE15	Tankang ('Paralysis Health')	Insertion: Indications:	(Anterior) 7 finger-widths above the lateral superior margin of the patella. Vertical, 1-2 cun. Paralysis of lower limb.
OLE16	Siqiang ('Four Strengths')	Insertion: Indications:	(Anterior) 4½ cun above the mid-point of the superior margin of the patella. Vertical, 1-2 cun. Paralysis of lower limb.
OLE17	Tanli ('Paralysis Erect')	Insertion: Indications:	(Anterior) 5 finger-widths above the lateral superior margin of the patella. Vertical, 1-2 cun. Paralysis of lower limb.
OLE18	Jianxi ('Strengthen Knee')	Insertion: Indications:	(Anterior) 3 cun above the mid-point of the superior margin of the patella, with the knee flexed. Vertical or slanted, 1-2 cun. Paralysis of lower limb; arthritis of knee.
OLE19	Tanfu ('Paralysis Recovered')	Insertion: Indications:	(Anterior) 3 finger-widths above the lateral superior margin of the patella. Vertical, 1-2 cun. Paralysis of lower limb.
OLE20	Kuangu ('Patella')	Insertion: Indications:	Two points, about 1½ cun to the left and right of St34 (Liangqiu). Vertical, 1-2 cun. Arthritis of knee; paralysis of lower limb.
OLE21	Zuluo ('Leg's Snare')	Insertion: Indications:	(Anterior) 3 cun above the superior margin of the medial condyle of the femur. Vertical, 1½-2½ cun. Irregular menses; puerperal fever; pain in the thigh and knee.
OLE22	Zuming ('Leg's Brightness')	Insertion: Indications:	(Anterior) 2 finger-widths above the superior margin of the medial condyle of the femur. Vertical, 1½-2½ cun. Arthritis of knee; puerperal fever.
OLE23	Dalun ('Big Wheel')	Insertion: Indications:	(Anterior) At the superior margin of the medial condyle of the femur. Vertical, 1½-2½ cun. Arthritis of knee; puerperal fever.
OLE24	Liaoliao ('Seam of the Seam')	Insertion: Indications:	(Anterior) On the prominence of the medial condyle of the femur. Slanted, 1-1½ cun. Irregular menses; abnormal uterine bleeding.

OLE25	Xixia ('Below Knee')		(Anterior) In the patella tendon, at the centre of the inferior border of the patella.
		Insertion:	Vertical, 1-1½ cun, or moxa.
		Indications:	Disorders of the knee-joint or surrounding tissues.
OLE26	Yinxia ('Below Abundance')		(Posterior) Midway between Bl50 (Chengfu) and Bl54 (Weizhong).
		Insertion:	Vertical, 1-2 cun.
		Indications:	Sciatica; low-back pain; paralysis of lower limb.
OLE27	Zhili ('Stand Erect')		(Posterior) 4½ cun above and ½ cun medial to Bl54 (Weizhong).
		Insertion:	Vertical, 1-2 cun.
		Indications:	Sequelae of poliomyelitis.
OLE28	Waizhili ('Outer Stand Erect')		(Posterior) 4½ cun above and 1½ cun lateral to Bl54 (Weizhong).
		Insertion:	Vertical, 1-2 cun.
		Indications:	Sequelae of poliomyelitis.
OLE29	Weishang ('Above the Commission')		(Posterior) 2 cun above Bl54 (Weizhong).
		Insertion:	Vertical, 1-2 cun.
		Indications:	Sequelae of poliomyelitis; pain in the leg.
OLE30	Shangyangquan ('Upper Hinge of Yang')		(Lateral) 1 cun above GB33 (Xiyangguan).
		Insertion:	Vertical, 1-2 cun.
		Indications:	Paralysis of lower limb; arthritis of knee.
OLE31	Lingbao ('Spirit's Treasure')		(Lateral) 6 cun above the lateral end of the popliteal crease.
		Insertion:	Vertical, 1-2 cun.
		Indications:	Mental illness; hysterical paralysis.
OLE32	Wuling ('Five Spirits')		(Lateral) 5 cun above the lateral end of the popliteal crease.
		Insertion:	Vertical, 1-2 cun.
		Indications:	Mental illness, hysterical paralysis.
OLE33	Silian ('Four Connections')		(Lateral) 4 cun above the lateral end of the popliteal crease.
		Insertion:	Vertical, 1-2 cun.
		Indications:	As OLE32.
OLE34	Yinwai 3 ('Yin's Commission')		(Lateral) 3 cun above the lateral end of the popliteal crease.
		Insertion:	Vertical, 1-2 cun.
		Indications:	As OLE32.
OLE35	Yinwai 2 ('Yin's Commission')		(Lateral) 2 cun above the lateral end of the popliteal crease.
		Insertion:	Vertical, 1-2 cun.
		Indications:	As OLE32.
OLE36	Yinwai 1 ('Yin's Commission')		(Lateral) 1 cun above the lateral end of the popliteal crease.
		Insertion:	Vertical, 1-2 cun.
		Indications:	As OLE32.

OLE37	Houyangguan ('Posterior Hinge of Yang')	Insertion: Indications:	(Lateral) 1 cun posterior to GB33 (Xiyangguan). Vertical, 1-2 cun. Pain in the knee; mental illness; paralysis of lower limb.
OLE38	Chenggu ('Complete Bone')	Insertion: Indications:	(Lateral) On the prominence of the lateral femoral condyle. Prick. Low-back pain; arthritis of knee.
OLE39	Xiwai ('Outside the Knee')	Insertion: Indications:	(Lateral) At the lateral end of the popliteal crease, slightly anterior to Bl53 (Weiyang). Vertical, ½-1 cun. Arthritis of knee; ulcerations on lower leg.
OLE40	Jixia ('Below the Basket')	Insertion: Indications:	(Medial) 2 cun below Sp11 (Jimen). Vertical, 1-2 cun. Paralysis of lower limb; weakness in adductor muscles.
OLE41	Jiejian ('Open Scissors')	Insertion: Indications:	(Medial) 4 cun above and 1½ cun posterior to Sp10 (Xeuhai). 1½ cun posterior to Jixia (OLE40). Vertical, 1-2 cun. 'Scissors Gait' due to cerebral palsy.
OLE42	Xinsheng ('New Life')	Insertion: Indications:	(Medial) 5 cun above the medial end of the popliteal crease. Vertical, 2-3 cun. Buerger's Disease.
OLE43	Shangxuehai ('Upper Sea of Blood')	Insertion: Indications:	(Medial) 3 cun above Sp10 (Xuehai). Vertical, 1-2 cun. Paralysis of lower limb; difficulty in leg-raising.
OLE44	Baichongwo ('Nest of a Hundred Insects')	Insertion: Indications:	(Medial) 1 cun above Sp10 (Xuehai). Vertical, 1-2 cun. Urticaria; eczema.
OLE45	Houxuehai ('Posterior Sea of Blood')	Insertion: Indications:	(Medial) 1½ cun posterior to Sp10 (Xuehai). Vertical, 1-2 cun. 'Scissors Gait' due to cerebral palsy.
OLE46	Shangququan ('Upper Crooked Spring')	Insertion: Indications:	(Medial) 3 cun above the medial end of the popliteal crease. Vertical, 2-3 cun. Buerger's Disease.
OLE47	Lishang ('Above the Measurement')	Insertion: Indications:	(Anterior) 1 cun above St36 (Zusanli). Vertical, 1-1½ cun. Sequelae of poliomyelitis.
OLE48	Erliban ('Two-and-a-half Measures')	Insertion: Indications:	(Anterior) ½ cun above St36 (Zusanli). Vertical, 1-2 cun. Acute gastro-enteritis.
OLE49	Liwai ('Outside the Measure')	Insertion: Indications:	(Anterior) 1 cun lateral to St36 (Zusanli). Vertical, 1-2 cun. Sequelae of poliomyelitis.

Anterior

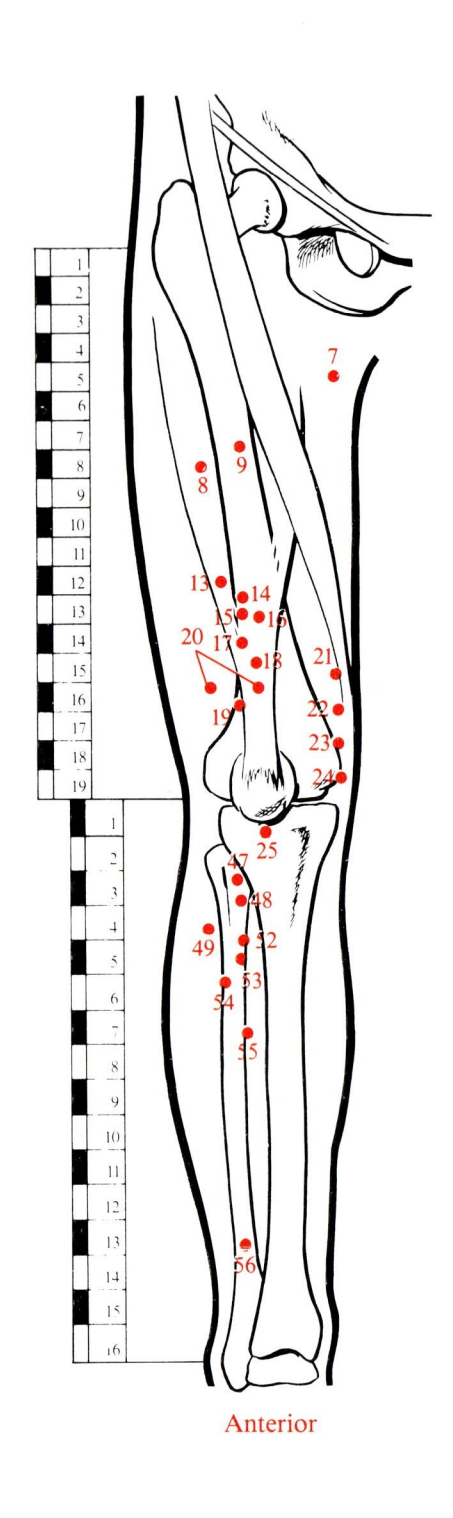

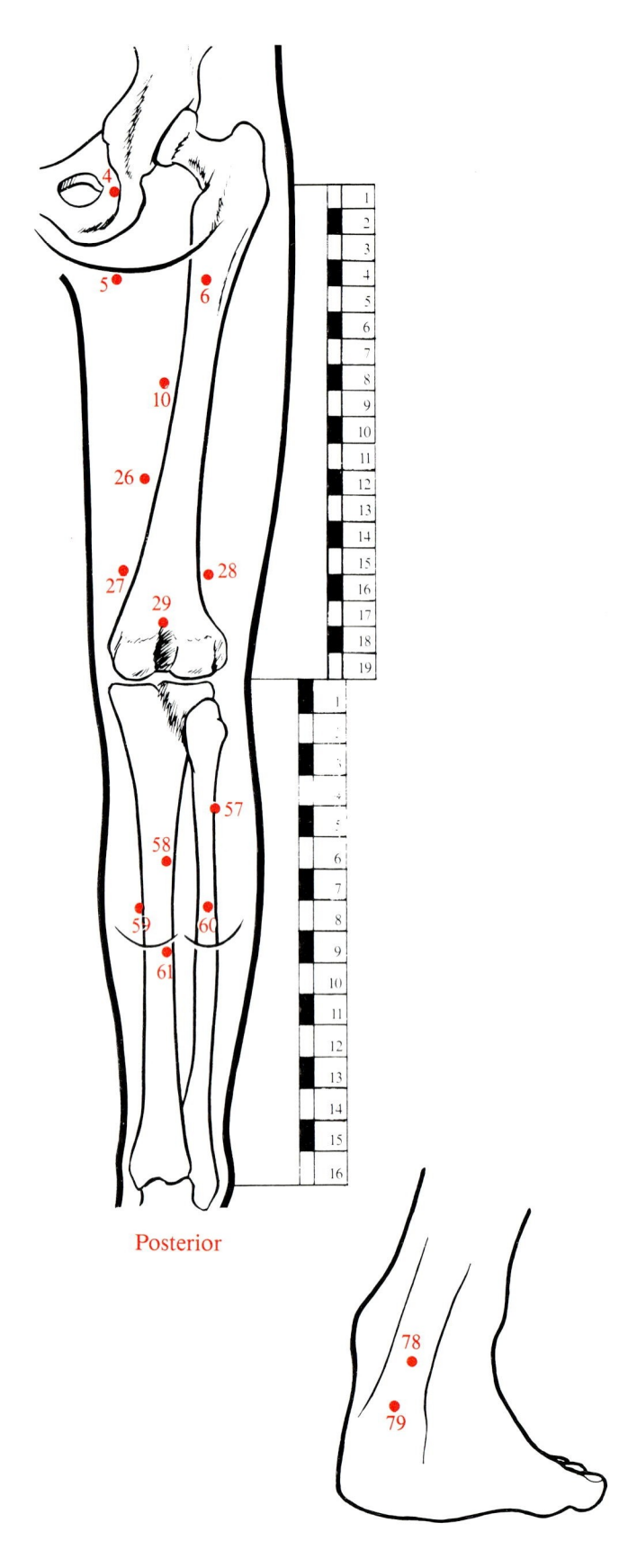

Posterior

64

65

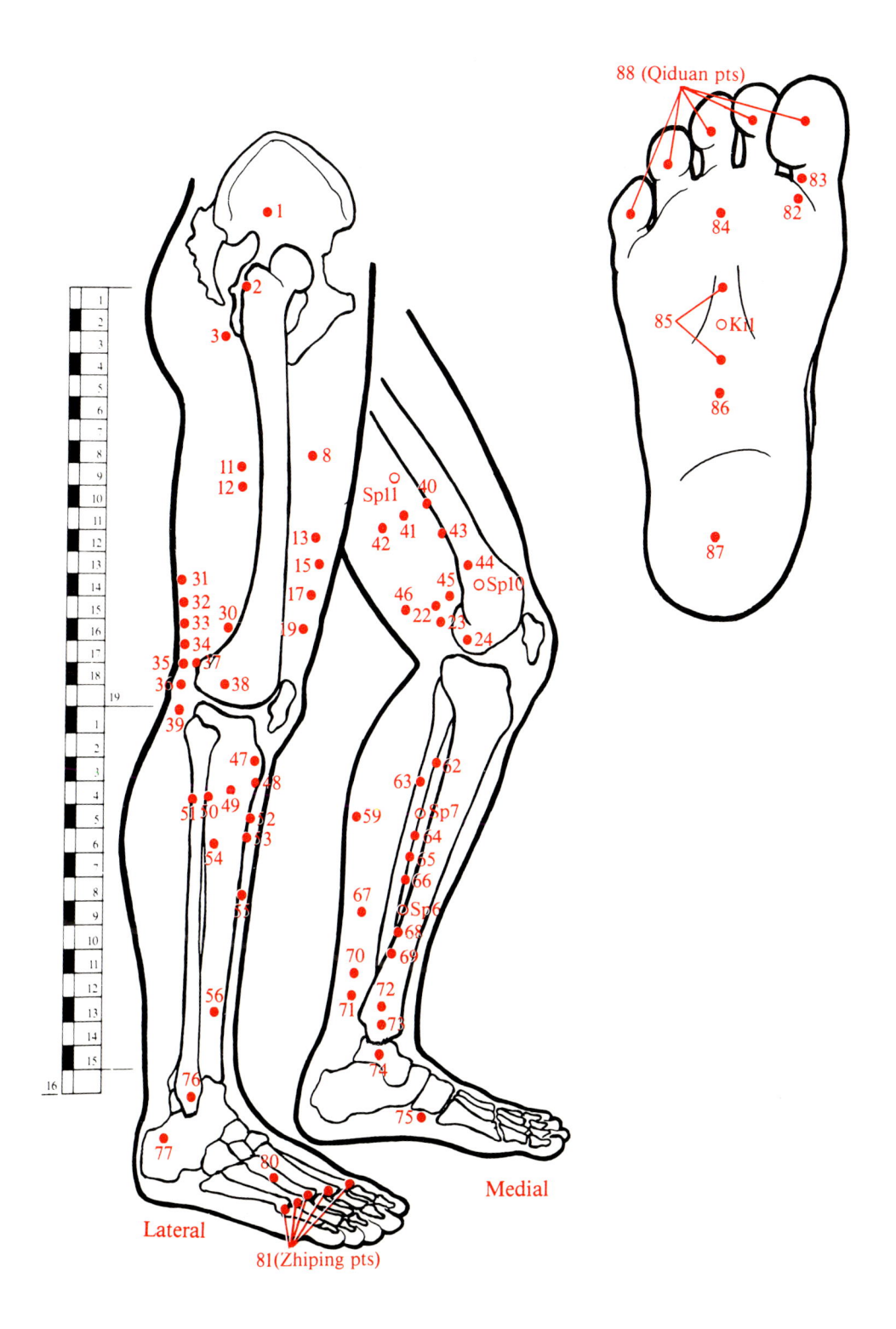

OLE50	Lingxia ('Below the Tomb')	Insertion: Indications:	(Lateral) 2 cun below GB34 (Yanglingquan). Vertical, 1-2 cun. Deafness; cholecystitis; biliary worms.
OLE51	Zuyicong ('Leg Benefit Hearing')	Insertion: Indications:	(Lateral) 3 cun below the capitulum of the fibula. Vertical or slanted, 1-1½ cun. Deafness; biliary worms.
OLE52	Wanli ('Ten Thousand Measures')	Insertion: Indications:	(Anterior) ½ cun below St36 (Zusanli). Vertical, 1½-2½ cun. Night blindness; optic nerve atrophy; ametropia; gastro-intestinal disorders.
OLE53	Zuzhongping ('Level with Mid-Leg')	Insertion: Indications:	(Anterior) 1 cun below St36 (Zusanli). Vertical, 1½-2½ cun. Mental illness; paralysis of lower limb.
OLE54	Sili ('Four Measures')	Insertion: Indications:	(Anterior) 1-1½ cun below St36 (Zusanli), 2 finger-widths lateral to the tibia. Vertical, 1½-2 cun. Poliomyelitis; paralysis.
OLE55	Zhitan 6 ('Treat Paralysis 6')	Insertion: Indications:	(Anterior) 1½ cun below Lanwei (LE6), 3½ cun below St36 (Zusanli). Vertical, 1-2 cun. Paralysis of lower limb.
OLE56	Jingxia ('Below the Tibia')	Insertion: Indications:	(Anterior) 3 cun above St41 (Jiexi) and 1 cun from the lateral border of the tibia. Vertical, ½-1 cun. Foot-drop; paralysis of lower limb.
OLE57	Weixia ('Below the Commission')	Insertion: Indications:	(Posterior) 4 cun below and 1½ cun lateral to Bl54 (Weizhong). Vertical, 1½-2½ cun. Sequelae to poliomyelitis; atrophy of gastrocnemius muscle.
OLE58	Chengjian ('Between Supports')	Insertion: Indications:	(Posterior) Midway between Bl56 (Chengjin) and Bl57 (Chengshan). Vertical, 1-2 cun. Sequelae of poliomyelitis.
OLE59	Jiuwaifan 2 ('Correct Outward Turning')	Insertion: Indications:	(Posterior) 1 cun medial to Bl57 (Chengshan). Vertical, 1-1½ cun. Sequelae of poliomyelitis with eversion of foot.
OLE60	Jiuneifan ('Correct Inward Turning')	Insertion: Indications:	(Posterior) 1 cun lateral to Bl57 (Chengshan). Vertical, 1-2 cun. Sequelae of poliomyelitis with inversion of foot.
OLE61	Xiachengshan ('Lower Support Mountain')	Insertion: Indications:	(Posterior) ½ cun below Bl57 (Chengshan). Vertical, 1½-2 cun. Tinea pedis.

OLE62	Dijian ('Ground Strength')	Insertion: Indications:	(Medial) 1 cun below Sp8 (Diji). Vertical, 1-2 cun. Eversion of foot.
OLE63	Lijimingandian ('Dysentery Sensitivity Point')	Insertion: Indications:	(Medial) 2/5ths of the distance from Sp9 (Yinlingquan) to the medial malleolus, at the most tender point. Vertical, 1-2 cun. Dysentery; sequelae of poliomyelitis.
OLE64	Jiaoyi ('Exchange Ceremony')	Insertion: Indications:	(Medial) 5 cun above the medial malleolus. Vertical, 1-2 cun. Irregular menses; leucorrhoea; beri-beri.
OLE65	Anmian 4 ('Peaceful Sleep')	Insertion: Indications:	(Medial) 1½ cun above Sp6 (Sanyinjiao). Vertical, ½-1½ cun. Insomnia; irritability.
OLE66	Yiniao ('Incontinence')	Insertion: Indications:	(Medial) 1 cun above Sp6 (Sanyinjiao). Vertical, ½-1 cun. Incontinence.
OLE67	Chengming ('Support Life')	Insertion: Indications:	(Medial) 3 cun above Ki3 (Taixi). Vertical, ½-1 cun. Mental illness; convulsions; oedema of lower leg.
OLE68	Jiuwaifan 1 ('Correct Outward Turning')	Insertion: Indications:	(Medial) ½ cun below Sp6 (Sanyinjiao). Vertical, 1-1½ cun. Sequelae of poliomyelitis with eversion of foot.
OLE69	Ganyandian ('Hepatitis Point')	Insertion: Indications:	(Medial) 2 cun above the medial malleolus. Vertical, 1-2 cun. Hepatitis; enuresis; dysmenorrhoea.
OLE70	Shaoyangwei ('Lesser Yang Link')	Insertion: Indications:	(Medial) Midway between Ki3 (Taixi) and Ki7 (Fuliu). Slanted, ½-1 cun. Chronic eczema of lower limbs; lupus; beri-beri; paralysis of leg.
OLE71	Shangxi ('Upper Stream')	Insertion: Indications:	(Medial) ½ cun above Ki3 (Taixi). Vertical, ½-1 cun. Eversion of foot.
OLE72	Zhizhuanjin ('Heal Turned Muscle')	Insertion: Indications:	(Medial) Centre of the upper border of the medial malleolus. Moxa. Spasm of gastrocnemius muscle; pain in ankle-joint; low-back pain.
OLE73	Neihuaijian ('Tip of Medial Malleolus')	Insertion: Indications:	(Medial) Tip of medial malleolus. Moxa. Muscle spasm of medial calf; toothache; tonsillitis.
OLE74	Taiyinqiao ('Greater Yin Heel')	Insertion: Indications:	(Medial) In depression at the lower border of the medial malleolus. Vertical, 3-5 fen. Irregular menses; menorrhagia; prolapsed uterus; female infertility.

OLE75	Chuqixue ('Vent Gas Orifice')	Insertion: Indications:	(Medial) ½ cun proximal to Ki2 (Rangu). Slanted, ½-1 cun. Distension in gastro-intestinal tract from oesophageal cancer.
OLE76	Waihuaijian ('Tip of Lateral Malleolus'	Insertion: Indications:	(Lateral) Tip of lateral malleolus. Prick. Toothache; paraplegia; severe headache; beri-beri.
OLE77	Xiakunlun ('Lower Kunlun Mountains')	Insertion: Indications:	(Lateral) 1 cun below Bl60 (Kunlun). Vertical, 3-5 fen. Arthritis; pain in low-back; paraplegia.
OLE78	Quanshengzu ('Spring at the Foot')	Insertion: Indications:	On the back of the heel, in the tendon, in the middle of the superior border of the calcaneum. Vertical, 2-3 fen. Oesophageal spasm; brain-disease; low-back pain.
OLE79	Nuxi ('Woman's Knees')	Insertion: Indications:	At the back of the heel, in the centre of the calcaneum. Vertical, 2 fen. Gingivitis; mental illness.
OLE80	Panggu ('Neighbouring Valley')	Insertion: Indications:	On the dorsum of the foot, 1 cun proximal to the web between the 3rd and 4th toes. Vertical, 3-5 fen. Sequelae of poliomyelitis.
OLE81	Zhiping ('Toe Level')	Insertion: Indications:	In the centre of the crease above the metatarsophalangeal joint on the dorsum of each toe. Slanted, 3-5 fen. Sequelae of poliomyelitis; paraplegia.
OLE82	Zhiwen ('Toe's Crease')	Insertion: Indications:	Plantar foot, in the centre of the crease between the hallux and the 1st metatarsal. Vertical 2-3 fen, or bleed. Hallux flexus.
OLE83	Muzhili-hengwen ('Transverse Crease of Big Toe')	Insertion: Indications:	Middle of plantar crease of hallux, distal to Zhiwen (OLE82). Vertical, 3-5 fen. Orchitis.
OLE84	Lineiting ('Within Inner Court')	Insertion: Indications:	Plantar foot, in the depression distal to the metatarsophalangeal joints of the 2nd and 3rd toes. Vertical, 3-5 fen. Painful toes; infantile convulsions; seizures.
OLE85	Qianhouyinzhu ('Hidden Pearls in Front and Back')	Insertion: Indications:	Two points, ½ cun proximal and distal to Ki1 (Yongquan). Slanted, 3-5 fen. Hypertension; pain in sole of foot; infantile convulsions.

OLE86	Zuxin ('Sole of Foot')	Insertion: Indications:	1 cun proximal to Ki1 (Yongquan). Vertical, ½-1 cun. Headache; plantar pain; abnormal uterine bleeding.
OLE87	Shimian ('Insomnia')	Insertion: Indications:	At centre of the plantar calcaneum. Vertical, 3-5 fen. Insomnia; local pain.
OLE88	Qiduan ('Qi's Extremity')	Insertion: Indications:	At the tip of each toe. Prick, or vertical 1-2 fen. Apoplectic coma; paralysis of toes; beri-beri; dorsum of foot red and swollen.

HAND NEEDLING — PALMAR POINTS

19.	Gastro-intestinal	Abdominal pain; gastro-enteritis.
20.	Heel	Sprained ankle.
21.	Common cold	Influenza; rhinitis.
22.	Hysteria	Emotional disturbance.
23.	Cough	Sore throat; chronic bronchitis.
24.	Oral ulcer	Pain in the mouth.
25.	Palpitation	Dizziness; chest discomfort.
26.	Nocturia (1)	Kidney diseases.
27.	Nocturia (2)	Bed-wetting.
28.	Polyhydrosis	Excessive sweating.
29.	Lung	Chronic cough; chest discomfort.
30.	Large Intestine	Vomiting; abdominal pain.
31.	Small Intestine	Diarrhoea.
32.	Heart	Palpitation.
33.	San-jiao	Lymphatic disorders.
34.	Spleen	Blood diseases.
35.	Liver	Jaundice; indigestion.
36.	Toothache	Toothache.

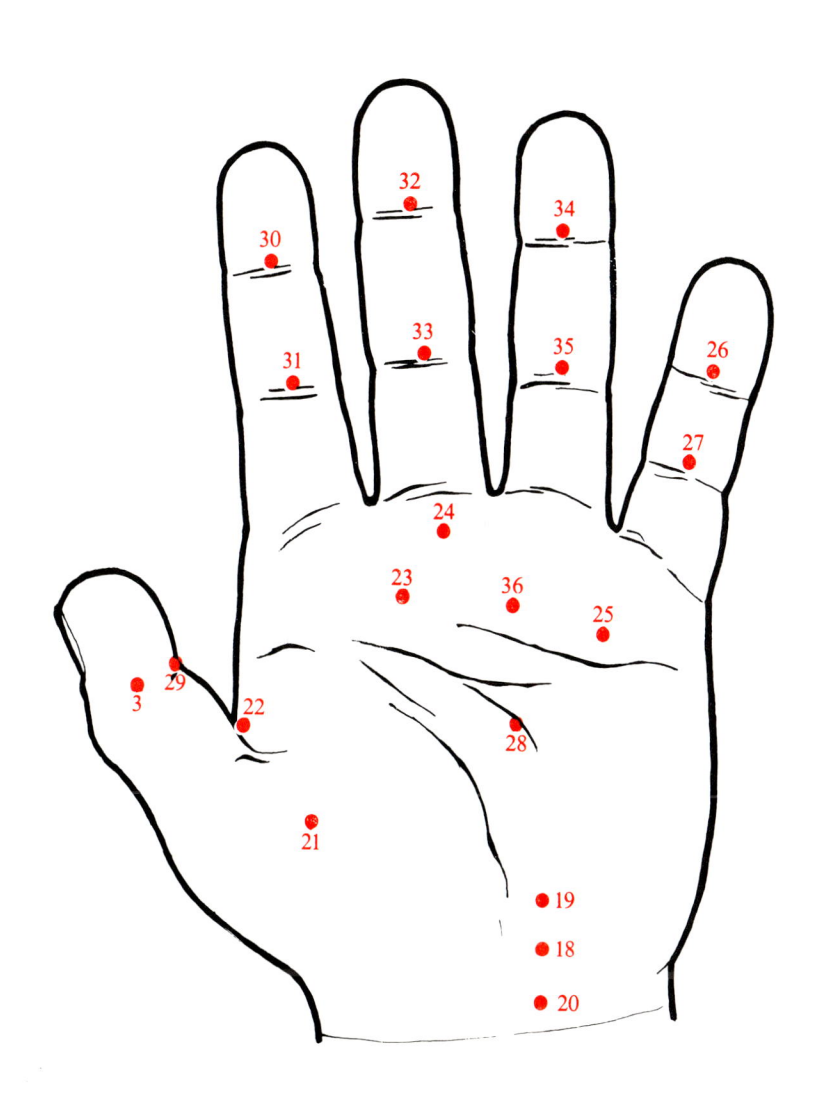

FOOT NEEDLING

Foot acupuncture is a not-very-well-known and often neglected aspect of the art, but can at times prove extremely effective.

The points are used bilaterally and are usually selected in pairs by matching points with similar or related indications, e.g. points 3 and 6 both have the indication of neurasthenia, and are thus a natural pair to select for this condition. In diseases of the extremities, of course, ipsilateral points may be used.

It is usual to use fairly strong stimulation, with the needles being retained for 3-5 minutes. The patient should be warned that these points are frequently painful, and the practitioner should be careful to avoid damage to the periosteum.

FOOT NEEDLING — PLANTAR POINTS

1. 1 cun distal to the posterior border of the heel, on the mid-line.
   Insertion: Vertical, ½ cun.
   Indications: Rhinitis; common cold; headache; sinusitis.
2. 3 cun distal to the posterior border of the heel, 1½ cun lateral to the mid-line.
   Insertion: Vertical, ½ cun.
   Indications: Intercostal neuralgia; pain or fullness in chest.
3. On the sole, midway between the medial and lateral malleoli.
   Insertion: Vertical or slanted distally, ½-1 cun.
   Indications: Neurasthenia; hysteria; insomnia; hypotension.
4. 1 cun medial to point No.3.
   Insertion: Vertical, ½ cun.
   Indications: Trigeminal neuralgia.
5. 4 cun distal to the posterior border of the heel, 1½ cun lateral to the mid-line.
   Insertion: Vertical, ½ cun.
   Indications: Sciatica; pain in low-back and leg.
6. 5 cun distal to the posterior border of the heel, 1 cun lateral to the mid-line.
   Insertion: Vertical, or slanted medially, ½-1 cun.
   Indications: Hysteria; neurasthenia; insomnia.
7. 5 cun distal to the posterior border of the heel, on the mid-line.
   Insertion: Vertical, ½ cun.
   Indications: Asthma; hepatitis; insomnia; incomplete maturation of brain.
8. 5 cun distal to the posterior border of the heel, 1 cun medial to the mid-line.
   Insertion: Vertical, 1-1½ cun.
   Indications: Diarrhoea; dysentery.
9. 1 cun distal to point 8.
   Insertion: Vertical, 1-1½ cun.
   Indications: Diarrhoea; dysentery.
10. 3 cun proximal to the mid-point of a line between the 4th and 5th toes.
    Insertion: Vertical, or slanted distally ½-1 cun.
    Indications: Sciatica; urticaria; pain in the shoulder.
11. 3 cun proximal to the mid-point of a line between the 3rd and 4th toes.
    Insertion: Vertical, or slanted medially 1-1½ cun.
    Indications: Dysmenorrhoea; gastro-enteritis.
12. 3 cun proximal to the mid-point of a line between the 1st and 2nd toes.
    Insertion: Vertical, 1 cun.
    Indications: Acute or chronic gastro-enteritis; spasm of the stomach.
13. 1 cun proximal to the middle of the crease under the 5th toe.
    Insertion: Vertical, or slanted distally ½-1 cun.
    Indications: Toothache.
14. In the middle of the crease below the 5th toe.
    Insertion: Slanted proximally, ½ cun.
    Indications: Incontinence; enuresis; frequency.
15. 1 cun proximal to the mid-point of a line between the 1st and 2nd toes.
    Insertion: Vertical, ½-1 cun.
    Indications: Toothache.

Plantar

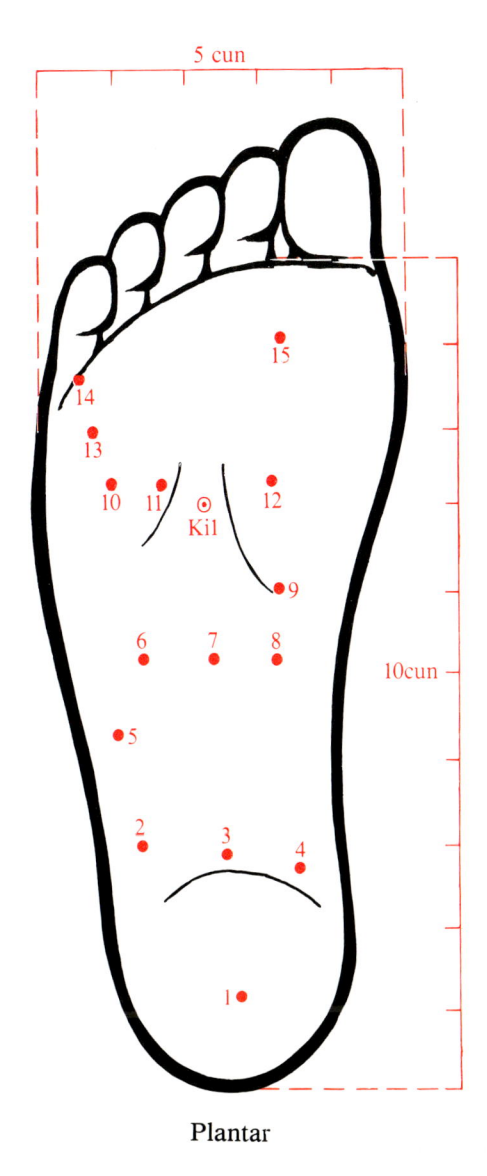

FOOT NEEDLING — DORSAL POINTS

16. ½ cun distal to St41 (Jiexi) in the depression lateral to it (lateral to the extensor tendon).
    Insertion: Slanted inferiorly or superiorly ½-1 cun, or join to point 17.
    Indications: Spasm of gastrocnemius muscle; low-back pain.
17. ½ cun distal to St41, in the depression medial to it (medial to extensor hallucis tendon).
    Insertion: As above.
    Indications: As above.
18. 2½ cun distal to St41 (Jiexi).
    Insertion: Vertical 1-5 fen, or prick.
    Indications: Angina pectoris; asthma; common cold.
19. 3 cun proximal to the mid-point of a line between the heads of the 2nd or 3rd metatarsals.
    Insertion: Vertical, or slanted upwards ½-1 cun.
    Indications: Gastric ulcer; duodenal ulcer; gastro-enteritis.
20. In the depression medial and distal to the base of the 1st metatarsal.
    Insertion: Vertical, 1-2 cun.
    Indications: Acute low-back strain.
21. 2 cun proximal to the mid-point of a line between the heads of the 3rd and 4th metatarsals.
    Insertion: Vertical, 1 cun.
    Indications: Torticollis; stiff neck.
22. Midway between GB41 (Zulingqi) and GB42 (Diwuhui).
    Insertion: Vertical, ½-1 cun.
    Indications: Sciatica; tonsillitis; parotitis.
23. Midway between Li2 (Xingjian) and Li3 (Taichong).
    Insertion: Vertical, or slanted proximally 1-2 cun.
    Indications: Tonsillitis; parotitis.
24. On the medial side of the proximal interphalangeal joint of the 4th toe.
    Insertion: Prick, 1-2 fen.
    Indications: Headache.
25. On the medial side of the proximal interphalangeal joint of the 3rd toe.
    Insertion: Prick, 1-2 fen.
    Indications: Headache.
26. On the medial side of the proximal interphalangeal joint of the 2nd toe.
    Insertion: Prick, 1-2 fen.
    Indications: Headache.
27. On the medial side of the extensor hallucis longus tendon, on the metatarsophalangeal joint.
    Insertion: Prick 1-2 fen, or shallow insertion.
    Indications: Eczema; urticaria; tonsillitis; parotitis.

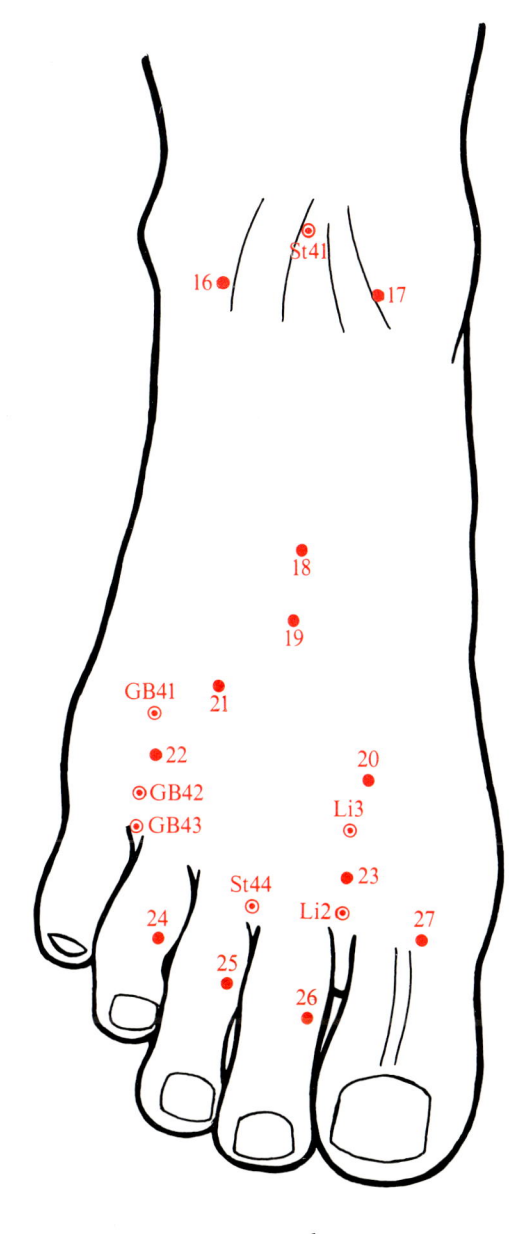

Dursal

FOOT NEEDLING — MEDIAL POINTS

28. Midway between Sp3 (Taibai) and Sp4 (Gongsun).
    Insertion: Horizontal, 1 cun.
    Indications: Epilepsy; hysteria; neurasthenia.
29. 1½ cun medial to St41 (Jiexi), in the depression above the navicular tubercle.
    Insertion: Vertical, ½ cun.
    Indications: Hypertension; tonsillitis; parotitis.
30. In the depression posterior and inferior to the navicular tubercle.
    Insertion: Vertical, 1 cun.
    Indications: Dysmenorrhoea; salpingitis; abnormal uterine bleeding.
31. 2 cun below the middle of the medial malleolus.
    Insertion: Vertical, 1 cun.
    Indications: Functional uterine bleeding.

FOOT NEEDLING — LATERAL POINTS

32. 1 cun above Bl60 (Kunlun).
    Insertion: Slanted, 1-2 cun.
    Indications: Headache; abdominal pain; sciatica.

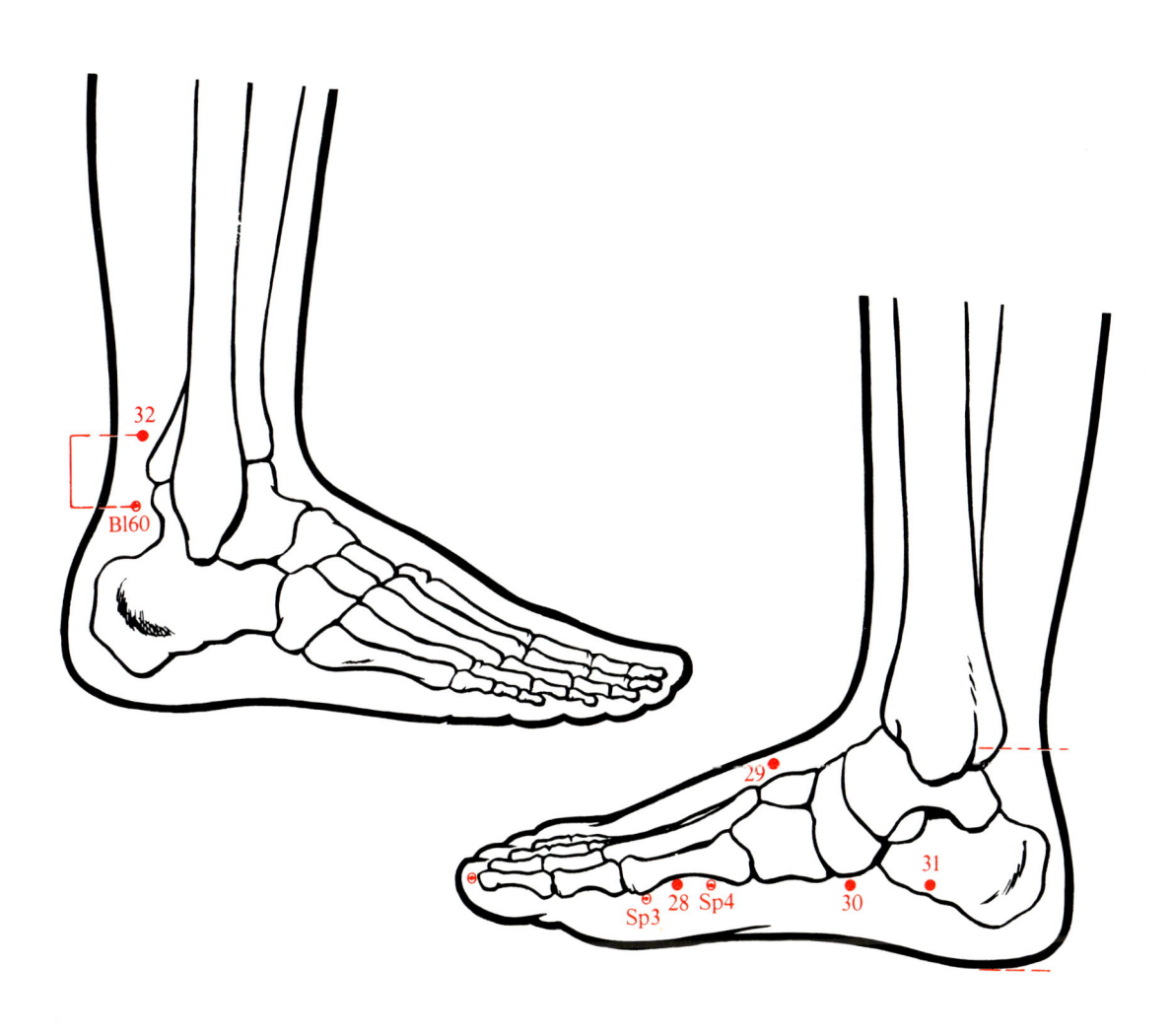

NOSE AND FACE NEEDLING

Nose needling, although nowadays primarily thought of as an adjunct to acupuncture analgesia, is of ancient origin and can be used also for therapeutic purposes. The nose was traditionally known as 'The Hall of Brightness', and the nose, the Zang-Fu, the four limbs, the bones and the circulation of Qi in the whole body were closely related, but especially the heart and the lungs. Needling nose points thus has a regulatory effect upon all the physiological processes.

Points are selected either upon the basis of their effect upon their pertained organ — i.e. Lung points to affect the lungs, Stomach points to affect the stomach, or upon their 5-Phase relationships — Kidney point to affect the bones, Lung point to affect the skin, etc. Spontaneous sensitivity is also an indication for their selection.

Distribution of Nose Points
There are 38 Nose points, including 8 single and 15 bilateral points. For convenience, 5 lines can be drawn on the nose region — one in the mid-line and two separated lines on each side, and with the exception of 'Testicle or Ovary' points, which are located on the outside of the first or mid-line, all the points are on these lines.

First line: Starts in the middle of the forehead and passes down the mid-line of the nose to the tip, with 8 points.

Second line: On both sides near the bridge of the nose. Start on the highest point of the bridge, and downwards to end at the lower border of the ala nasae. 5 points on each side.

Third line: Starts from the inner end of the eye-brow, down along the groove of the nose 1-2cm lateral from the second line, and ends on the termination of the wing of the nose. 9 points on each side.

Needle Insertion
1-1½ inch 30 gauge filiform needle. Insert vertically to the subcutis, then at an angle of 20° slanted along the subcutis, or piercing ½-1 cun. In order to avoid pain in a sensitive area, be careful not to penetrate the cartilage and do not 'force' the needle.

Directions of Insertion:

1. First line: Kidney and External Genitalia points — straight insertion.
   Other points — Downwards slanting insertion.

2. Second line: Slant downwards in the direction of the Third line.

3. Third line: Ear point — slanting insertion towards Heart point.
   Chest point — slanting insertion towards Nipple point.
   Other points — slant downwards.

NOSE AND FACE NEEDLING
Point Distribution

First Line

Head and Face	In the middle of the forehead, on the midline of a line connecting the centre between the eyebrows and the natural margin of the hair.
Pharynx and Larynx	Middle of the line connecting 'Head and Face' and 'Lung'.
Lung	Midway between the inner ends of the eye-brows.
Heart	Midway between the internal canthii.
Liver	Below the most prominent part of the bridge of the nose, the crosspoint between the line connecting the two zygomatic bones and the midline of the nose. Midway between 'Heart' and 'Spleen'.
Spleen	Midline of upper border of tip of nose. Midway between 'Heart' and 'External Genitalia'.
Kidney	Midway between 'Spleen' and 'External Genitalia'.
External Genitalia	On the tip of the nose.
(Testicle/Ovary	Bilateral, lateral to the tip of the nose, and on the inner border of the alae nasae).

Second Line

Gall Bladder	Below the medial angle of the orbit, lateral to 'Liver'.
Stomach	Below 'Gall Bladder', lateral to 'Spleen'.
Small Intestine	At upper ⅓ of alae nasae, below 'Stomach'.
Large Intestine	Middle of alae nasae, below 'Small Intestine'.
Bladder	On end border of alae nasae, below 'Large Intestine'.

Third Line

Ear	Inner end of the eye-brow.
Chest	Below 'Ear', above the orbital fossa.
Mammary Gland	Medial side of the internal canthus, below 'Chest'.
Neck and Back	Medial aspect of internal canthus, below 'Mammary Gland'.
Lumbar vertebrae	Medial aspect of zygomatic bone, on level of 'Liver'.
Upper Limb	Level of upper margin of tip of nose, same level as 'Spleen', below 'Lumbar vertebrae'.
Groin	Upper margin of alae nasae, below 'Upper Limb'.
Knee and Leg	Outer side of middle of alae nasae on nasolabial groove, below and slightly lateral to 'Groin'.
Toes	Below 'Knee and Leg', on same level as 'Bladder'.

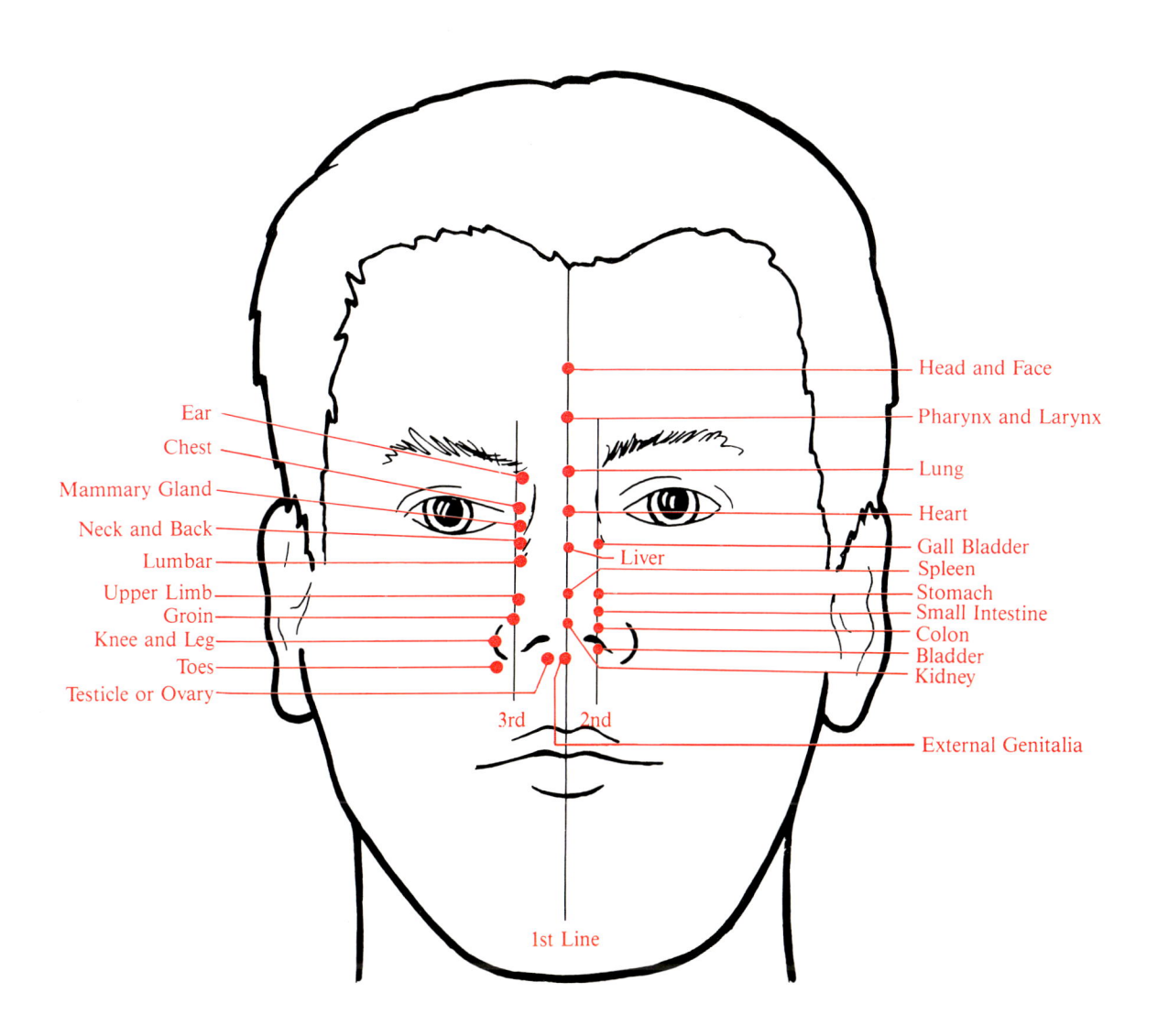

NOSE NEEDLING ANALGESIA

For purposes of analgesia the points are selected as in the opening paragraph, but in every case the point 'Lung' is invariably used, together with what is known as the 'operative field' point, this latter being the corresponding representative points of the area to be operated upon. For the paired points one or both points may be used.

1. *Operations upon the neck*
   Subtotal thyroidectomy: Lung, Pharynx and Larynx,
   Fistulectomy of thyroglossal duct: Lung, Pharynx and Larynx.
2. *Operations upon the chest*
   Pericardiostomy and drainage: Lung, Heart.
   Dilatation of bicuspid valve: Lung, Heart.
   Thoracotomy: Lung, Thorax.
   Radical mastectomy: Lung, Thorax, Mammary Gland.
3. *Operations upon the abdomen*
   Perforated peptic ulcer: Lung, Stomach.
   Gastrectomy: Lung, Stomach.
   Splenectomy: Lung, Spleen.
   Cholecystectomy: Lung, Gall Bladder.
   Intestinal resection: Small Intestine piercing through to Large Intestine.
   Appendectomy: Lung, Small Intestine piercing through to Large Intestine.
   Hernioraphy: Lung, External Genitalia.
   Caesarean section: Lung, Ovary, External Genitalia.
   Hysterectomy: Lung, Ovary, External Genitalia.
   Oophorectomy: Lung, Ovary, External Genitalia.
   Fallopian ligation, Salpingectomy: Lung, Ovary, External Genitalia.
   Cystolithotomy, ureterolithotomy: Lung, Ear, Bladder, External Genitalia.
4. *Operations upon the Lower Limbs*
   Extirpation of elephantiasis: Lung, Knees, Leg piercing through to Toes.
   Open reduction of femoral fracture: Lung, Groin.
   Amputation of Lower Limb: Lung, Groin.

FACE NEEDLING

Uterus and Bladder	In the philtrum, junction of middle and upper thirds.
Inside of Thigh	5 fen lateral to the oral angle. (Same point as St4 Dicang).
Shoulder	On the upper border of the malar bone, vertically below the external canthus.
Arm	Posterior to 'Shoulder', on the upper border of the zygomatic arch.
Hand	Below 'Arm', on the lower border of the zygomatic arch.
Back	In front of the tragus, between the inner side of the tragus and the mandibular joint.
Thigh	⅓ the distance from the ear-lobe to the angle of the mandible.
Knee	⅓ the distance from the angle of the mandible to the ear-lobe.
Patella	(Same point as St6 Jiache). In the depression above the angle of the mandible.
Lower Leg	On the upper border of the mandible, anterior to the mandibular angle.
Foot	Anterior to 'Lower Leg', vertically below the external canthus, on the upper border of the mandible.
Kidney	Vertically below Taiyang on the level of the ala nasi.
Umbilicus	On the cheek, 7 fen below 'Kidney'.

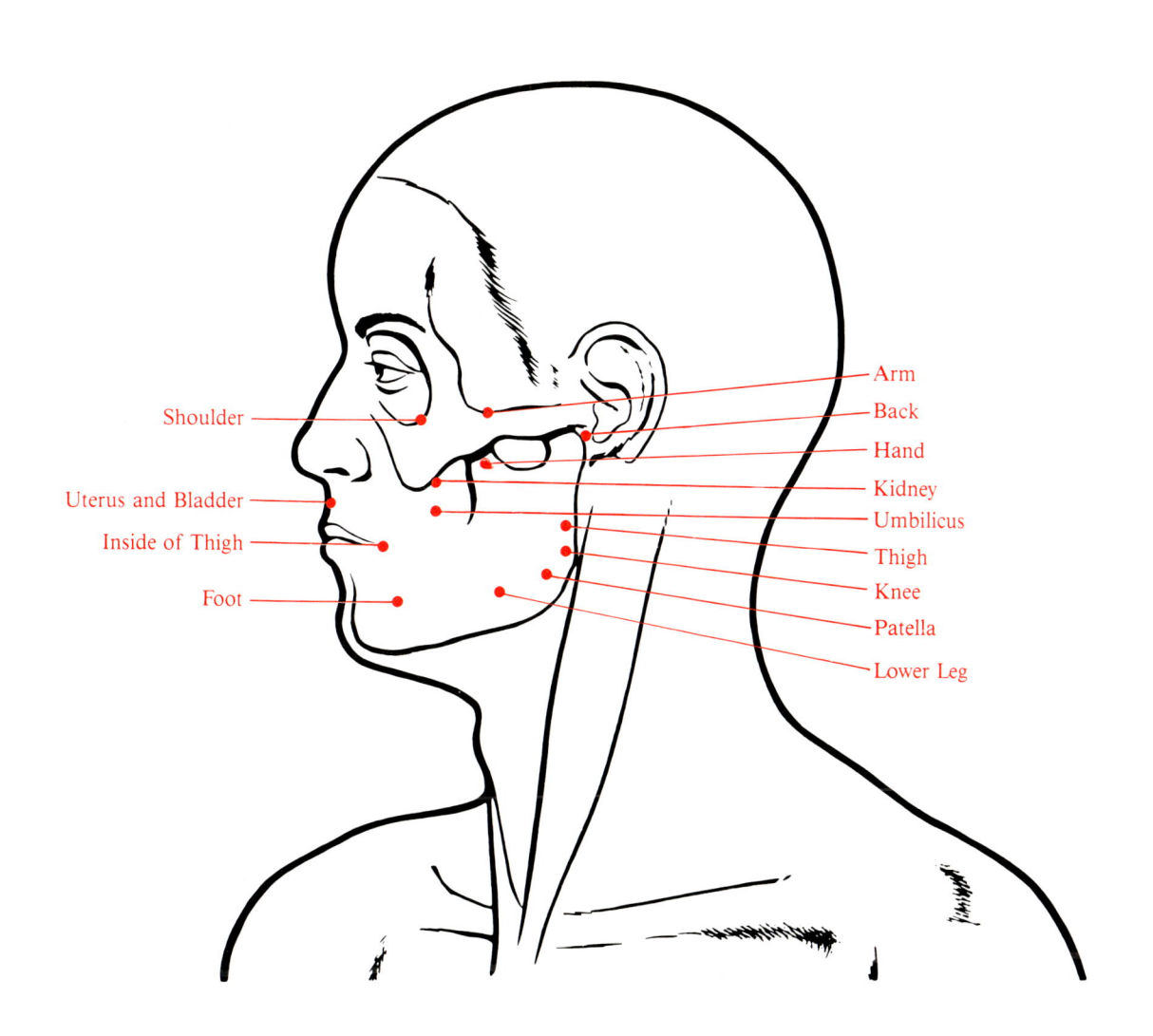

HEAD NEEDLING

Head or scalp needling is possibly the most important of all the various acupuncture techniques which have evolved since the Ming dynasty (ending 1644). It took its rise from the work of Dr Jiao Shen-fa, a neurologist working in Ji Shan People's Hospital during the Cultural Revolution, and was originally evolved for treating intractable cases of hemiplegia by needling the area on the scalp that is related to the motor areas of the cerebral cortex. Other areas were later discovered by utilizing the same basic principle, leading to the mapping-out of the sensory, visual, speech and similar areas.

It is particularly useful for the treatment of the various forms of motor and sensory impairment which can so often prove difficult to resolve using the standard body or auricular therapy, but organ dysfunctions can also respond to stimulation of the appropriate areas — in these conditions head-needling is usually used only when the condition has failed to respond to the more normal approaches.

For motor and sensory conditions, bearing in mind the decussation of the pyramidal tracts, it is usual to treat the opposite side, whilst bilateral conditions are treated bilaterally.

The usual strict aseptic precautions have to be observed, and it is preferable to use a fairly thick needle of 26 or 28 gauge, 2½ to 3 inches long. The needle is inserted at a 15° angle to the skin, and then gently rotated subcutaneously to the required distance, usually about 1½ inches. The needle should be rotated to obtain Da Qi, and then rotated with a wide amplitude at a frequency of 200 per minute for two to three minutes. The needle is then left *in situ* for five to ten minutes, rotated again, and then withdrawn slowly, the point of insertion being cleaned with dry sterilized cotton-wool to prevent bleeding and infection.

Electro-stimulation may also prove effective, again at a frequency of 200 per minute (or slightly over 3Hz), for about 20 to 30 minutes.

The sensation experienced by the patient should be a feeling of warmth, or occasionally numbness or tingling, in the affected area or limb, whilst to prevent needle-sickness it is advisable for the patient to be treated either prone or supine, if possible.

In China, patients are treated daily for 10-16 days, rested for 5-7 days, and the course is then repeated if necessary. In the West this frequency of treatment is less easy to attain, but bi-weekly treatment is preferable, and certainly no longer than a week between treatments. With the greater gap, the over-all period of treatment is naturally greatly increased.

Locating the Areas
In mapping-out the areas, there are two standard, essential guidelines to establish:

1. The Antero-Posterior Midline, connecting the mid-point between the two eye-brows and the lower border of the external occipital tuberosity.

2. The Eye-Brow/Occiput line, connecting the mid-point of the eye-brow with the tip of the external occipital tuberosity.

All other stimulation areas are mapped from these two lines, and are usually linear with a width of about 3 millimetres.

1. *Motor Area* (Corresponds to the anterior central gyrus).
   The upper point is 0.5 centimetre posterior to the mid-point of the A/P line.
   The lower point is where the Eye-Brow/Occipital line crosses the anterior margin of the natural hair line on the temple. (If the hair is absent, take a vertical line upwards from the mid-point of the zygomatic arch. The lower point of the Motor Area is on the Eye-Brow/Occipital line 0.5 centimetres anterior to this vertical.)

The Motor Area is divided into five parts, the upper $\frac{1}{5}$th being the motor area of the lower limbs and trunk, the middle $\frac{2}{5}$ths the motor area of the upper limbs, and the lower $\frac{2}{5}$ths (also known as 'Speech 1') the motor area for the face and speech organs (corresponds to Broca's area and the inferior frontal gyrus).

2. *Sensory Area* (Corresponds to the post-central gyrus of the parietal lobe).
   Is a line parallel to and 1.5cm posterior to the Motor Area. This area is also divided into five parts: Upper $\frac{1}{5}$th sensory to the lower limbs, trunk and neck, middle $\frac{2}{5}$ths sensory to the upper limbs, and the lower $\frac{2}{5}$ths sensory to the head and face.
3. *Chorea.* 1.5cm anterior to the Motor Area.
4. *Vaso-Vagal.* 1.5cm anterior to Chorea.
5. *Inner Ear.* (Corresponds to the middle portion of the superior temporal gyrus). 1.5cm above the apex of the ear, 4cms long.
6. *Speech 3.* (Corresponds to the posterior portion of the superior temporal gyrus). This line overlaps Inner Ear by 2cms and continues posteriorly to a total of 4cms.
7. *Functional Area.* (Corresponds to the supramarginal gyrus of the parietal lobe). Starts at the intersection of a vertical line from the end of Speech 3, and a horizontal line from the parietal tuberosity. It extends downwards for 3cms at an angle of 40° from the vertical on both sides of the vertical line.
8. *Speech 2.* (Corresponds to the angular gyrus of the parietal lobe). Is a vertical line 3cms long starting from 2cms below the parietal tuberosity.
9. *Leg and Foot.* On the vertex of the head, parallel to the A/P line at 1cm distance from it, starting 1cm anterior to GV20 (Paihui) and ending 3cms posterior to this point.
10. *Visual Area.* (Corresponds to the upper and lower border of the calcarine fissure of the occipital lobe). Parallel to the A/P line at 1cm distance from it, extending 4cms upwards from the inion.
11. *Equilibrium.* (Corresponds to the cerebellar hemisphere). Parallel to the A/P line, at 3.5cms distance from it, extending 4cms downwards from the inion.
12. *Stomach Area.* Take a straight line from the centre of the pupil vertically upwards to the hair margin. The prolongation of this line for 2cms above the hair margin is the Stomach Area.
13. *Thoracic Area.* Is on a vertical line mid-way between Stomach Area and the A/P line, from 2cms below to 2cms above the hair-line.
14. *Genitalia.* Is a vertical line 1.5cm posterior to Stomach Area, 2cms long.
15. *Liver and Gall Bladder.* The straight line extending for 2cms below the Stomach Area.
16. *Intestines.* The straight line extending 2cms below the Genitalia area,.

Indications
1. Upper Motor: Paralysis or paresis of contralateral lower limb and trunk.
   Middle Motor: Paralysis or paresis of contralateral upper limb.
   Lower Motor: Contralateral facial paralysis: slurred speech; motor aphasia; aphonia; excessive salivation.
2. Upper Sensory: Pain or numbness, all abnormal sensations, of contralateral lower limb, trunk and neck. Occipital headache.
   Middle Sensory: All sensory defects in contralateral upper limb.
   Lower Sensory: Facial paraesthesia; trigeminal neuralgia; right or left sided migraine; arthritis of temporo-mandibular joint.
3. Chorea: Has similar regional sub-divisions as the Motor and Sensory areas. For all involuntary movements — Parkinsonism, tics, facial hemi-spasm, chorea, blepharospasm, senile tremor.
4. Vaso-Vagal: Generalized oedema; high or low blood-pressure; cerebral oedema; oedema from hypertension or from paralysis of the limbs.
5. Inner Ear: Tinnitus, Menière's Disease, vertigo, deafness.
6. Speech 3: Loss of speech, sensory aphasia.
7. Functional: Apraxia and loss of function.
8. Speech 2: Alexia and word aphasia.

9. Leg and Foot: Pain, numbness or paralysis of the lower limbs; uterine prolapse, nocturia; acute lumbago.
10. Visual Area: Poor sight due to cortical visual disturbances; colour blindness.
11. Equilibrium: Loss of balance, vertigo, caused by cerebellar disorders.
12. Stomach: Abdominal pain above the umbilicus; gastric disorders; general malaise.
13. Thoracic: Bronchial asthma; dyspnoea; palpitations; pain in thoracic area.
14. Genitalia: Functional uterine bleeding; ejaculatio praecox. All genital conditions with a nervous basis. Also uterine prolapse when used in conjunction with motor-sensory 'foot' area.
15. Liver and Gall Bladder: Liver and Gall Bladder dysfunction; pain or discomfort in the epigastrium and right hypochondrium.
16. Intestines: Intestinal dysfunction.

Note: Head Needling is most suitable for:
    Head injuries; cerebro-vascular accident; concussion; Parkinsonism; Menières's syndrome.

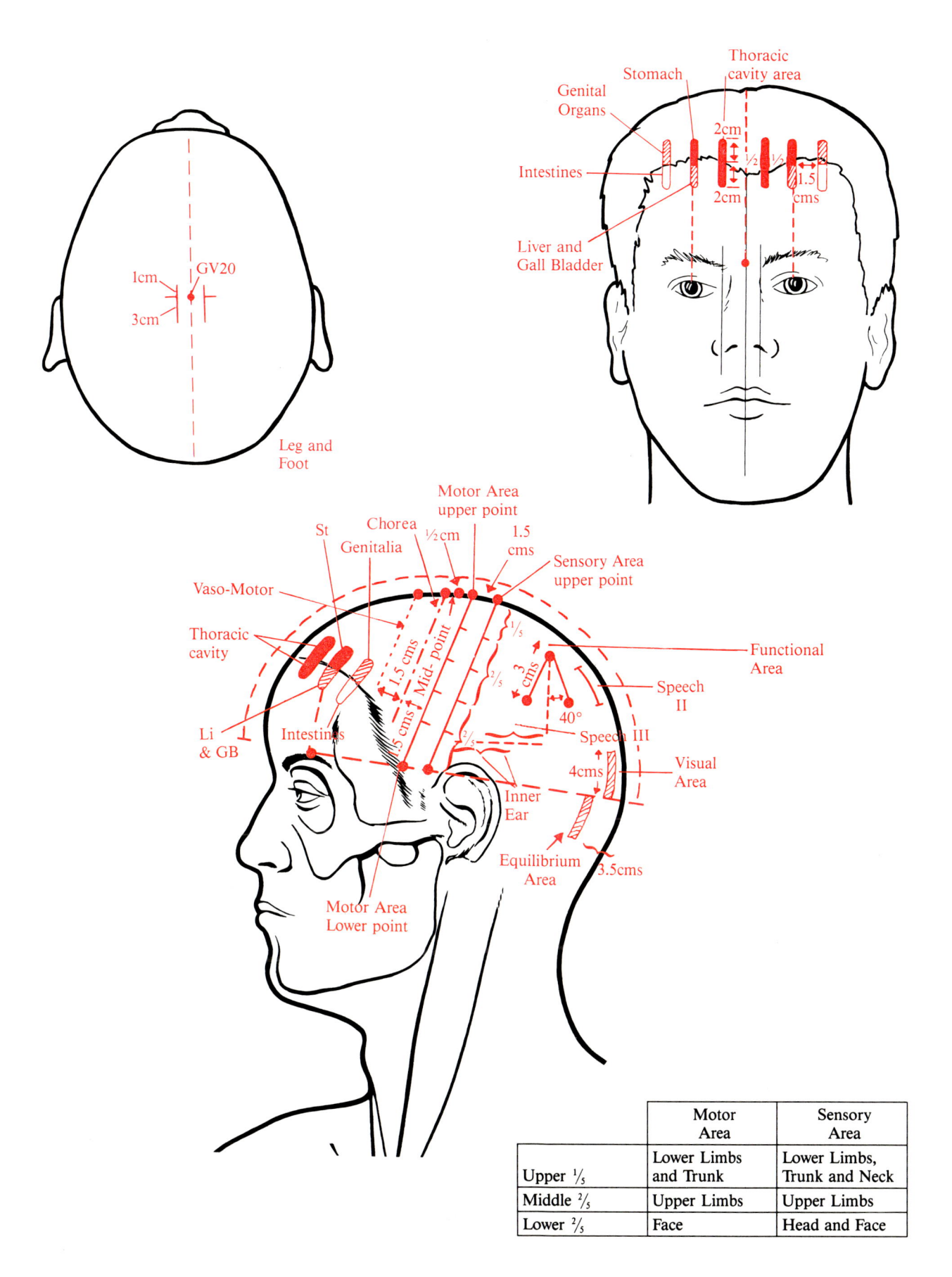

	Motor Area	Sensory Area
Upper 1/5	Lower Limbs and Trunk	Lower Limbs, Trunk and Neck
Middle 2/5	Upper Limbs	Upper Limbs
Lower 2/5	Face	Head and Face

95

KOU LIANG TECHNIQUES AND COLLECTIVE LOCI

Kou Liang means 'Two Mouths', and refers to the technique of piercing through from one point to join it up with another, thereby combining the actions of the two points and enhancing their effect. Collective Loci refers to the use of a particular 'grouping' of points to produce an increased action.

Both of these techniques are used to great effect in present day China, and listed here are some of the more commonly used prescriptions:

1. Co20 → Bitong (FA8): All forms of rhinitis; paranasal sinusitis.
2. GB20 → GB20: Common cold; influenza; headache; pain in the neck; psychosis; eye-diseases.
3. TH21 → GB2
   St7 → SI19
   Add: Shen-chi (¼ of way down the posterior ear-crease)
   TH18, TH17,
   Ehr-Ting (in the cavum concha, 2 fen lateral to the auditory meatus) — Deafness; tinnitus; otitis media.
4. Taiyang → GB8
   GB20 → GB8 — Stubborn migraine; pain and stiffness in neck and nape.
5. GB4 → GB7 (bilateral) — Headache; migraine; vertigo; neurasthenia; facial paralysis; spasm; Menière's disease; polyneuritis.
6. GV23 → GV20
   GV18 → GV20 — Intractable headache.
7. CV15 → CV21 — Bronchitis; bronchial asthma; TB; chest pain; hysteria; epilepsy; heart failure; hypotension; tachycardia.
8. CV12 → CV13 — Peptic ulcer; acute and chronic gastritis; cardiac spasm; vomiting; constipation; diarrhoea; indigestion.
9. Bl21 → Bl20 — Peptic ulcer; gastroptosis; haemorrhagic disease; neurogenic vomiting; indigestion; hepato-splenomegaly; pancreatitis; hepatitis.
10. Bl38 → SI15 (Subcutaneously with thick 1mm needle) — Diseases of the eye.
11. GV14 → GV9 — Epilepsy; hysteria; cerebral paralysis; psychosis; neurasthenia; furunculosis; neuro-dermatitis; palpitations; bronchitis; asthma; back-pain; intercostal neuralgia.
12. GV8 → GV5 — Visceral disorders (Liver, Gall-Bladder, Spleen, Stomach, etc.).
13. GV4 → GV3 — Genito-urinary system; sciatica; paralysis of lower limbs.
14. Lu9 → Lu8 (bilaterally) Or, vertically into Lu9, withdraw, insert to Lu8. — Bronchitis.
15. HC7 → HC4 — Heart failure; disturbance of peripheral circulation; shock; collapse; syncope; hypotension; tachycardia; Menière's disease; cloudiness of brain; epilepsy; vomiting.
16. Ht7 → Ht4 — Insomnia; epilepsy; psychosis; palpitations; paroxysmal

		tachycardia; heart failure; hypertension; hypotension; somnambulism; excessive dreaming; neurasthenia; hysteria.
17.	HC6 → TH5	Pain in carpal joint; wrist-drop; sequelae of CVA; hysterical paralysis; angina pectoris; polyneuritis; sore throat; tinnitus.
18.	Co11 → Ht3, with another vertically into HC3.	Paralysis of upper limb; pain in shoulder and elbow joints; pain and swelling in throat; hypertension; high fever; swelling of thyroid gland; urticaria.
19.	TH10 → TH12	Paralysis of upper limb; difficulty in raising shoulder; pain in shoulder and elbow joints.
20.	Co4 → HC8 (2-3 cun)	Tremor of hands and feet; polyneuritis; sweating in palm; salivation; sequelae of CVA; hysterical paralysis; psychosis; headache; toothache.
21.	St32 oblique → St31	Indigestion in children; stomach-ache; splenomegaly; nephritis; paralysis of lower limbs.
22.	GB34 → Sp9	Pain in knee joint; sciatica; sequelae of CVA; arrhythmia; equinovarus; cholecystitis; biliary ascariasis; intercostal neuralgia; constipation.
23.	GB39 → Sp6	Equinovarus; polyneuritis; stiff neck; diseases of ankle joint and tissues; hemiplegia; nephritis; enteritis.
24.	Bl61 → Bl58	Hemiplegia; epilepsy; lumbago; pain in leg; sciatica; abdominal pain; oedema; intestinal tympanitis; constipation; enuresis; retention of urine; dysmenorrhoea; menstrual abnormalities; amenorrhoea; leucorrhoea; polyneuritis; talipes valgus.
25.	GB34 → GB38	Hemiplegia; sequelae of poliomyelitis; osteo-arthrosis of knee; pain in lower limb; cystitis; urethritis.
26.	Weishang (OLE29) → Bl50	Hemiplegia; sequelae of poliomyelitis; pain in thigh; polyneuritis.
27.	GB30 → Bl50	Sciatica.
28.	Bl57 → Bl54	Hemiplegia; rheumatoid arthritis; numb cold leg; polyneuritis; spasm of calf muscle; intestinal tympanitis; constipation; retention of urine; enuresis.
29.	St38 → Bl57	Inflammation of the shoulder joint; peripheral neuritis; haemorrhoids; sciatica.
30.	Ki5, insert to 5 fen, withdraw, then → Ki7	Hyperhydrosis; dysfunction of sweat glands (including hypohydrosis); retention of urine; enuresis; nephritis; cystitis; urethritis; talipes valgus.
31.	Bl60 → Ki3	Local; menstrual difficulties; pharyngitis; tinnitus; headache; lumbago.
32.	St7 → St6 St7 → St2 St4 → St6 St4 → St2 Can add TH17, Co4.	Facial paralysis; facial spasm.

Collective Loci

33.	Anmian (HN3) bilaterally, with GV14.	Neurasthenia; insomnia; epilepsy; hysteria.
34.	St25 bilaterally, with Zhixie (CA8)	Diarrhoea; enteritis; dysentery.

35.	Zigong (CA9) with CV3	Spermatorrhoea; impotence; leucorrhoea; dysmenorrhoea; uterine prolapse; frequency; enuresis.
36.	Hu-Kung (2.6 cun lateral to CV6) with CV4	Infertility; adnexitis; ovarian tumour; orchitis.
37.	4 points each 1 cun above, below, and on both sides of CV8.	Dysentery; enteritis; indigestion; food-poisoning.
38.	Dingchuan (DL 3) bilaterally with GV14.	Upper respiratory tract infection; cough; asthma; high fever.
39.	Co15, with Jian-Jian (1 cun above anterior axillary crease) and Jian-Hou (1½ cun above posterior axillary crease).	Pain in shoulder and back; frozen shoulder.
40.	Xiyan points (LE 5) with GB34.	Pain and sprain of knee-joint.
41.	GV24 → GV20, Shen-chi (¼ way down posterior ear-crease), Sp6 → GB39; Li2 → Li3.	Hypertension.
42.	CV15, 17, 22, 23, Dingchuan, GV14, Lu9, Co6.	Acute tracheitis; chronic bronchitis and brochial asthma.
43.	CV5, Sp13, Li-Chung (5 cun below tibial tuberosity and 1 cun lateral to anterior margin of tibia) Li2 vertically, then → to Li3	Lower abdominal pain; appendicitis; dysmenorrhoea.
44.	CV10, 12, 14; St21; Co9; Bao-Jian (3 cun below tibial tuberosity, 3 fen lateral to anterior margin of tibia).	Acute and chronic gastritis; gastric spasm; enteritis; dysentery.
45.	CV3, 4, 9; St28; Sp6; Li2 → Li3	Renal oedema.
46.	CV10, 12, 14; St21; Co9; Ki16; Bao-Jian (see 44)	Gastric and duodenal ulcers.

REPERTORY

Abbreviations used in this repertory:
Special Points:
- Face — FA
- Head and Neck — HN
- Chest and Abdomen — CA
- Dorsal and Lumbar — DL
- Arm and Hand — AR
- Leg and Foot — LE

Other non-meridial points:
- Face — OFA
- Mouth — M
- Head and Neck — OHN
- Chest and Abdomen — OCA
- Dorsal and Lumbar — ODL
- Arm and Hand — OAR
- Leg and Foot — OLE
- Hand Needling — Hand
- Foot Needling — Foot
- Kou-Liang — K-L

(Nose, Face and Head needling have not been repertorized as the names of the areas correlate to the conditions for which they are used.)

General and Infectious Conditions
Visceral disorders generally: (Li, GB, St, Sp, etc): K-L12.
Infantile malnutrition syndrome: AR15
Adnexitis: OCA22, K-L36.
Lymphatic disorders: Hand 33.
Emaciation unit Thirst: M2, M3.
General debility: ODL15, ODL59.
Exhaustion: AR16.
Heat-stroke: AR16, OFA18, OAR48.
High fever: AR16, OAR49, K-L38.

Shock: OAR34.
Oedema — general: OCA27, K-L24.
   " — pedum: OLE67.
   " — renal: K-L45.
Malaria: OAR41, ODL22.
Beri-beri: OLE64, OLE70, OLE76, OLE88.
Pertussis: AR15.
Diabetes: ODL21, ODL22, OLE14.
Influenza: OAR49, Hand 21.
T.B. — Scrofula: HN9, ODL8, OAR9, OAR26, K-L7.
    Inguinal lymph-glands: CA10.
    Lung: ODL15, ODL59.
    Intestines: ODL35.
Lupus: OLE70.

Endocrine Glands
Hyperthyroidism: OHN5.
Swelling of Thyroid: K-L18.
Goitre: OHN5, OHN8, OHN35, OHN36, OAR5.
Pituitary adenoma: OHN33.

Neurological Conditions
Sequelae of brain disease: OHN30, OHN31.
Sequelae of CVA: K-L20, K-L22.
Sequelae of poliomyelitis: AR3, AR4, AR9, LE3, LE10, LE11, ODL42, OLE5, OLE6, OLE7, OLE9, OLE10,
   OLE11, OLE12, OLE27, OLE28, OLE29, OLE47, OLE49, OLE 54, OLE57, OLE58, OLE63, OLE80,
   OLE81, K-L25, K-L26.
   Affecting hip: OLE2.
Paraplegia: DL8, ODL38, OLE1, OLE3, OLE11, OLE76, OLE77, OLE81.
Hemiplegia: AR1, AR5, AR7, LE3, OHN13, OHN27, OHN32, OAR3, OLE1, OLE7, OLE11, OLE12,
   K-L23, K-L24, K-L25, K-L26, K-L28.
Paralysis: Facial: FA9, FA10, OFA6, OFA13, OFA14, OFA16, OFA17, K-L5, K-L32,
    Eye-muscles: OFA8.
    Upper arm: OAR23.
    Upper limbs: DL4, AR6, OHN8, OAR5, OAR20, OAR28, OAR29, OAR31, OAR32, K-L18, K-L19.
    Wrist-drop: AR6, K-L17,
    Hands (Palms): OAR10.
    Lower limbs: CA13, DL6, LE1, LE2, LE6, LE7, LE8, ODL36, ODL40, ODL46, ODL47, ODL53,
      OLE4, OLE8, OLE13, OLE14, OLE15, OLE16, OLE17, OLE18, OLE19, OLE20, OLE26,
      OLE30, OLE37, OLE40, OLE43, OLE53, OLE55, OLE56, OLE70, K-L13, K-L21.
    Weakness of leg adductors: CA10, OLE40.
    Difficulty in leg-raising: OLE43.
    Gastrocnemial spasm: ODL50.
    Gastrocnemial atrophy: OLE57.
    Foot-drop: LE6, LE9, LE10, LE11, OLE56.
    Toes: OLE58.
    'Scissor's Gait' due to cerebral palsy: OLE41, OLE45.
    Respiratory muscles: OHN11.
Hysterical paralysis: OLE31, OLE32, OLE33, OLE34, OLE35, OLE36, K-L11, K-L17, K-L20.
Tremors of hands and feet: K-L20.
Tremors: OHN8.

Brain
Incomplete maturation of cerebral cortex: OHN34, Foot 7.
Hydrocephalus: OHN28.
Brain diseases: ODL2, OLE78.
Apoplexy: ODL7.
Apoplectic coma: OLE88.
Slurred speech: HN6.
Aphasia: M1, OHN1, OHN7.
Mutism: HN6, OHN1, OHN7.
Polyneuritis: K-L5, K-L17, K-L20, K-L23, K-L24, K-L26, K-L28.
Peripheral neuritis: LE12, LE13, K-L29.
Spinal cord (meningitis): DL1a, ODL1.
Lateral sclerosis: OHN13, ODL1.
Myelitis: ODL1, ODL58.

Mental Conditions
Generally: HN2, OAR1, OAR2, OAR31, OLE 31, OLE32, OLE33, OLE34, OLE35, OLE36, OLE37, OLE53, OLE67, OLE79.
Emotional disturbances: Hand 22.
Mania: DL11, OHN12.
Psychosis: OFA15, OFA19, OHN34, OAR17, OAR40, K-L2, K-L20.
Hysteria: AR7, OHN12, ODL9, OAR40, Foot 3, Foot 6, Foot 28, K—L7, K-L11, K-L16, K-L33.
Schizophrenia: HN3, HN4.
Neurasthenia: OHN12, OHN26, Foot 3, Foot 6, Foot 28, K-L7, K-L11, K-L16, K-L33.
Epilepsy: DL9, ODL4, ODL27, Hand 3, Foot 28, K-L7, K-L11, K-L15, K-L16, K-L24, K-L33.
Convulsions: OFA15, OFA19, OHN26, OHN34, ODL27, OAR17, OAR40, OLE67, OLE84.
    " (Infantile): FA1, OAR10, OLE84, OLE85.
Retardation from encephalitis: LE10, OHN12.
Idiocy after brain-disease: OHN19.
Progressive loss of memory: OFA19, OAR17.
Amnesia: LE10.
Irritability: ODL19, OLE65.
Restlessness: HN4.
Lassitude: LE10.
Insomnia: FA1, HN2, HN3, HN4, OFA10, ODL19, OAR17, OLE65, OLE87, Foot 3, Foot 6, Foot 7, K-L16, K-L33.
Hypersomnia: OHN19.

Neuralgia: Supra-orbital: FA2.
        Trigeminal: FA10, OFA13, OFA16, Hand 13, Foot 4.
        Forearm: AR7, AR10.
        Femoral nerve: LE2.
        Intercostal: OCA2, OCA3, OCA8, ODL12, ODL14, ODL20, ODL21, ODL22, Hand 3, Foot 2, K-L11, K-L22.
To stimulate nerves of pelvic plexus: ODL56.

Musculo-Skeletal
Head: OAR36.
Stiff-neck: HN8, HN9, AR12, AR13, AR14, OHN10, OHN32, ODL4, OAR13, OAR39, OAR43, Foot 21, K-L2, K-L4, K-L23.

Torticollis: Foot 21.
Cervical syndrome: Hand 14.
Dorsal area: DL1(b), DL3, ODL11.
Shoulder: DL3, DL4, AR1, AR2, AR3, AR5, AR8, AR14, ODL10, OAR1, OAR2, OAR3, Hand 5, Foot 10, K-L18, K-L19, K-L29, K-L39.
Back of shoulder: ODL7;
Scapula: ODL9.
Arms: Hand 10.
Forearm: AR7, AR10, OAR6, OAR28.
Elbow: OAR21, OAR25, OAR27, K-L18, K-L19.
Wrist: AR11, OAR35, Hand 18, K-L17.
Fingers: AR12, AR13, AR15, AR16, OAR43, OAR44.
 " (Numb): OAR14, OAR37.
Chest pain: OCA7, Hand 8, Hand 25, Hand 29, Foot 2, K-L7.
Costal chondritis: OCA3.
Atrophy of pectoralis major muscle: OCA5.
Pigeon-breast: OCA4.
Lumbar area: DL7, DL10, ODL31, ODL36, ODL41, ODL43, OAR30, OAR36, Hand 11, K-L24, K-L31.
Acute low-back strain: Foot 20.
Lumbo-sacral area: DL8, LE2, ODL36, ODL39, ODL50, OLE8, OLE26, OLE38, OLE72, OLE77, OLE78, Hand 1, Foot 5, Foot 16, Foot 17, K-L11.
Sacro-Iliac: ODL44.
Hip: Hand 12.
Lower limbs: ODL44, OAR36, OLE29, K-L24, K-L25, K-L26.
Knee: LE4, LE5, LE8, OLE8, OLE13, OLE18, OLE20, OLE21, OLE22, OLE23, OLE25, OLE30, OLE37, OLE38, OLE39, K-L22, K-L25, K-L40.
Spasm of gastrocnemius muscle: OLE72, Foot 16, Foot 17.
Spasm of medial calf: OLE73.
Ankle: OLE72, Hand 2, Hand 20, K-L23.
Eversion of foot: OLE59, OLE62, OLE68, OLE71, K-L22, K-L23, K-L24, K-L30.
Inversion of foot: OLE60.
Foot: LE12, LE13.
Dorsum of foot: OLE88.
Sole of foot: OLE85, OLE86.
Plantar heel: OLE87.
Toes: LE12, LE13, OLE84, OLE88.
Hallux flexus: OLE82.
Sciatica: DL8, DL10, LE1, LE2, LE8, ODL39, ODL47, ODL53, OAR43, OLE4, OLE5, OLE6, OLE10, OLE12, OLE26, Hand 1, Hand 12, Foot 5, Foot 10, Foot 22, Foot 32, K-L13, K-L22, K-L24, K-L27, K-L29.
Spondylitis: DL1(a), DL6, ODL1, ODL58.
Inflammation of vertebral ligaments: DL6.
Arthritis: OLE77.
Rheumatoid arthritis: K-L28.
Hernia: CA6, CA7.

Headaches
General: FA1, HN2, AR12, AR13, LE12, LE13, OFA7, OFA11, OHN9, OAR38, OLE76, OLE86, Hand 7, Hand 16, Foot 1, Foot 24, Foot 25, Foot 26, Foot 32, K-L2, K-L5, K-L6, K-L20, K-L31.
Migraine: FA3, HN3, AR14, OFA6, OFA8, OFA20, K-L4, K-L5.
Unilateral: Hand 8.

Vertex: OHN26.
Lateral or Vertex: FA3.
Frontal: Hand 6.
Occipital: HN8, OHN22, Hand 10.
Neurotic: OHN12.

Sinusitis, Rhinitis, etc.
General: OAR25, Hand 17, Foot 1.
Frontal: FA2, OFA7, OFA10.
Nasal: FA7, FA8, K-L1.
Rhinitis: FA1, FA7, FA8, OFA12, OFA13, OFA14, ODL3, Hand 11, Hand 21, Foot 1, K-L1.
Common cold: ODL4, OAR48, Hand 21, Foot 1, Foot 18, K-L2.
Epistaxis: OAR45, Hand 15.

Respiratory Tract
Nasal polypii: FA7, FA8.
Nasal furuncle. OFA12, OFA14.
Sore throat: HN8, AR12, AR13, AR14, OAR42, OAR44, Hand 23, K-L17, K-L18.
Tonsillitis: HN5, M1, ODL5, OAR12, OAR14, OAR46, OAR49, OLE73, Hand 10, Hand 13, Foot 22, Foot 23, Foot 27, Foot 29.
Pharyngitis, laryngitis: HN5, HN6, OFA18, OHN3, OHN20, ODL5, OAR10, Hand 13, K-L31.
Tracheitis: K-L42.
Disease of vocal cords: OHN2, OHN3, OHN6.
Bronchitis: DL1(b), AR11, OCA3, OCA6, ODL4, ODL6, ODL11, ODL12, ODL14, ODL15, ODL18, ODL59, OAR35, Hand 23, K-L7, K-L11, K-L14, K-L38, K-L42.
Asthma: DL3, AR11, M5, OCA2, OCA6, ODL4, ODL6, ODL12, ODL15, ODL18, ODL59, OAR12, OAR35, Foot 7, Foot 18, K-L11, K-L38.
Brochial asthma: K-L7, K-L42.
Cough: HN9, DL3, OCA2, Hand 29, K-L38.
Apnoea: OHN11.
Haemoptysis: ODL20.
Pneumonia: DL1(b), ODL11, ODL20.
Pleurisy: DL1(b), OCA8, ODL11, ODL18.
T.B. of lung: ODL15, ODL59.
Hiccups: OCA10, OAR45, Hand 10.
Spasm of diaphragm: M2, OHN11.

Circulatory
Haemorrhagic disorders: ODL32.
Blood diseases: Hand 34.
Anaemia: ODL51, ODL59.
Heart trouble generally: ODL12.
Rheumatic heart disease: ODL37, OAR4, OAR11.
Valvular disease of heart: OAR7.
Heart failure: OAR34, K-L7, K-L15, K-L16.
Arrhythmia: K-L22.
Palpitations: HN4, AR6, AR9, OFA10, OAR4, OAR7, OAR11, Hand 32, K-L11, K-L16.
Tachycardia: K-L7, K-L15, K-L16.
Bradycardia: OHN19.
High blood pressure: DL2, Foot 29.

Hypertension: FA1, AR1, OHN18, OAR24, OAR39, OLE85, K-L16, K-L18, K-L41.
Low blood pressure: DL2.
Hypotension: Foot 3, K-L15, K-L16.
Angina pectoris: Foot 18, K-L17.
Buerger's disease: ODL45, OLE42, OLE46.
Poor circulation in legs: CA10, K-L15.
Ulcerations on lower-leg: OLE39.
Cold feet: ODL47.

Genito-Urinary Tract
Tract generally: ODL17, K-L13.
Nephritis: OCA12, OCA14, ODL17, ODL31, K-L21, K-L23, K-L30.
Pyelonephritis: CA9.
Kidney diseases: Hand 26.
Cystitis: CA9, OCA21, ODL36, K-L25, K-L30.
Urethritis: K-L25, K-L30.
Gonococcal urethritis: ODL49.
Incontinence: OCA25, OLE66, Foot 14.
Incontinence due to paraplegia: OCA23, OCA26, ODL52, ODL54, ODL57.
Retention of urine: CA8, OFA16, K-L24, K-L28, K-L30.
Enuresis: CA12, OLE69, Hand 27, Foot 14, K-L24, K-L28, K-L30, K-L35.
Nocturia: ODL33.
Frequency: Foot 14, K-L35.
Renal Oedema: K-L45.
Oedema Pedum: OLE67.
General Oedema: OCA27, K-L24.

Gastro-Intestinal Disorders
Lack of appetite: OCA12.
Belching: OCA14.
Mouth: Parotitis: FA9, HN2, OFA21, OAR49, Foot 22, Foot 23, Foot 27, Foot 29.
    Excess phlegm: OHN4.
    Salivation: HN6.
    Pain in mouth: Hand 24.
    Toothache: AR12, AR13, AR17, LE12, LE13, OFA29, OHN9, OAR6, OAR14, OAR15, OAR38,
      OLE73, OLE76, Hand 13, Hand 36, Foot 13, Foot 15, K-L20. (Lower Jaw — OFA17, OAR33).
    Pain in gums: ODL13.
    Gingivitis: OLE79.
    Mouth ulcers: FA9, M4, Hand 24.
    Ulcers on gums: M4.
    Stomatitis: HN6, M1, OHN1, OAR10, OAR16.
    Glossitis: M1.
    Swollen tongue: OHN2.
    Tongue feels heavy: M3.
    Paralysis of tongue: M5, OHN1.
Indigestion: CA1, LE6, OCA12, OCA13, OCA14, OCA15, OCA27, ODL28, Hand 35, K-L8, K-L9, K-L21, K-L37.
Indigestion (Infantile): AR15.
Food-poisoning: K-L37.
Abdominal pain, gastralgia, stomach ache: CA3, DL5, AR11, AR14, LE12, LE13, OCA7, ODL13, ODL23,

ODL28, OAR35, OAR38, OLE9, Hand 6, Hand 19, Hand 30, Foot 32, K-L21, K-L24.
Gastritis: OCA13, K-L8, K-L44.
Gastric disorders: ODL21, ODL25, ODL33.
Gastric hyperacidity: CA2.
Peptic ulcer: OCA12, K-L8, K-L9.
Gastric ulcer: DL5, OCA13, ODL30, Foot 19, K-L46.
Duodenal ulcer: ODL30, Foot 19, K-L46.
Spasm of stomach: OCA27, OAR39, Foot 12, K-L44.
Prolapsed stomach: CA1, CA3, CA4, K-L9.
Vomiting: M1, OHN4, ODL13, OAR45, Hand 3, Hand 30, K-L9, K-L15.
Vomiting and diarrhoea: OAR47.
Gastro-enteritis: OCA27, ODL28, ODL33, OAR48, OLE48, OLE52, Hand 6, Hand 19, Foot 11, Foot 12, Foot 19.
Gastro-enteritis (Infantile): OAR46.
Enteritis: CA8, OCA14, OCA15, OCA17, ODL28, ODL31, ODL35, ODL49, OLE9, K-L23, K-L34. K-L37, K-L44.
Intestinal dysfunction: CA7, ODL33.
Borborygmus: CA11.
Tympanitis: K-L24, K-L28.
Distension of gastro-intestinal tract from oesophageal cancer: OLE75.
T.B. of intestines: ODL35.
Schistosomiasis: OCA11, ODL29, ODL56.
Diarrhoea: CA2, Hand 31, Foot 8, Foot 9, K-L34.
    " (Infantile): OCA19.
Dysentery: CA8, OCA15, OLE63, Foot 8, Foot 9, K-L34, K-L37, K-L44.
Constipation: OFA16, OCA17, K-L22, K-L24, K-L28.
Constipation due to paraplegia: OCA16.
Appendicitis: CA9, LE6, K-L43.
Peritonitis: OCA17.
Anal prolapse: AR10, ODL28, ODL35, ODL55.
Haemorrhoids: AR10, ODL33, ODL35, OAR6, K-L29.
Blood in stool: ODL35.
Perianal pain: Hand 9.

Liver, Gall Bladder, Spleen and Pancreas
Liver disorders: ODL25, ODL26.
Pain in liver area: OCA9.
Hepatomegaly: OCA9, ODL31, ODL34.
Hepatitis: ODL14, ODL16, ODL22, OLE69, Foot 7, K-L9.
Gall Bladder and bile-duct: LE7, ODL14, ODL25, ODL26.
Cholecystitis: OLE7, OLE50, K-L22.
Biliary colic: Hand 8.
Biliary worms: OLE50, OLE51, K-L22.
Jaundice: Hand 35.
Splenomegaly. ODL16, ODL31, ODL34, K-L9, K-L21.
Pancreatitis: ODL16, K-L9.

Gynaecology and Obstetrics
Mastitis: OCA8, OAR7.
Breast tumour: OCA1.

Pelvic inflammatory conditions. CA5, CA9.
Lower abdominal pain: CA6, CA11, CA13, K-L43.
General gynaecological conditions: DL7, DL8, K-L31.
Ovarian hyperplasia: ODL34.
Ovarian tumour: K-L36.
Salpingitis: Foot 30.
Uterine prolapse: CA6, CA7, CA9, OCA24, ODL55, OLE74, K-L35.
Dysmenorrhoea: CA9, OFA15, OLE69, Foot 11, Foot 30, K-L24, K-L35, K-L43.
Abnormal uterine bleeding: OCA25, ODL48, OLE24, OLE86, Foot 30.
Functional uterine bleeding: Foot 31.
Menorrhagia: OCA12, OCA21, ODL41, OLE74.
Irregular menses: CA9, LE12, LE13, OCA17, OCA18, OCA22, ODL49, OLE21, OLE24, OLE64, OLE74, K-L24.
Amenorrhoea: ODL34, K-L24.
Leucorrhoea: ODL48, OLE64, K-L24, K-L35.
Puerperal leucorrhoea: OCA21.
Puerperal fever: OLE21, OLE22, OLE23.
Difficult labour: ODL50.
Miscarriage: OCA19.
Infertility: CA5, OCA25, K-L36.
Sterility: CA9, OCA21, OLE74.

Male Sexual Disorders
Impotence: OCA20, K-L35.
Premature ejaculation: OCA20.
Spermatorrhoea: ODL34, K-L35.
Pain in penis: OCA22.
Orchitis: CA9, OCA21, OCA22, OLE83, K-L36.
Scrotal eczema: OCA20.

Skin and Dermatology
Skin diseases generally: OHN17.
Urticaria: ODL7, ODL47, OAR22, OLE44, Foot 10, Foot 27, K-L18.
Eczema: OLE44, Foot 27.
Eczema of legs: OLE70.
Eczema of scrotum: OCA20.
Allergic dermatitis: OAR22.
Neuro-dermatitis: K-L11.
Pruritis: OAR22.
Scabies: OAR41.
Tinea pedis: OLE61.
Carbuncle: OAR8, OAR26.
Ulcerations of lower leg: OLE39.
Hyper- and hypo-hydrosis: K-L30.
Hyperhydrosis: AR1, Hand 28, K-L30.

Sense Organs
Eyes: Palpebritis: OFA8.
　　　Weak sight: OFA11.
　　　　Myopia: FA4, HN2, OFA8.

Ametropia: FA5, FA6, OFA1, OFA2, OFA3, OFA3d, OFA4a, OFA4b, OFA9, OLE52.
Hypermetropia: HN2.
General eye-troubles: OFA6, OAR20, OAR41, OAR42, OAR44, OAR47, K-L2, K-L10.
Blurred vision: OFA7.
Optic nerve troubles: FA4, FA5, FA6, HN2, OFA1, OFA2, OFA3, OFA3b, OFA3c, OFA5, OLE52.
Optic atrophy: ODL24.
Retinitis: ODL24.
Retinitis pigmentosa: FA4, OFA3, OHN22.
Retinochoroiditis: OFA3b.
Retinal haemorrhage: OFA5.
Dacryocystitis: OFA3b.
Eyes water: OFA1, OFA2.
Glaucoma: FA4, OFA3d, OHN18, OHN22.
Corneal opacity, cataract: FA2, FA4, HN2, OFA3, OFA3d, OFA4a, OFA4b, OFA20, OHN21, OAR35.
Macula corneae: OFA3b.
Corneal ulcer: OFA3a.
Keratoleukoma: FA5, FA6.
Eyes sore, red, swollen: FA3.
Conjunctivitis: FA2, OFA5, OFA11, OFA18, OFA20, OHN 17, OAR46, Hand 4.
Nebula: OFA3a, OFA3b, OFA4, OFA4a, OAR19.
Pannus: OAR19.
Squint: FA4, OFA1, OFA2, OFA3, OFA3c.
Night blindness: OAR18, OAR46, OLE52.
Hordeolum: OHN17.
Nose: Nasal polypii: FA7, FA8.
Nasal furuncle: OFA12, OFA14.
Hyposmia: OFA13, ODL3.
Epistaxis: OAR45, Hand 15.
Ears: General: OFA29.
Otitis media: K-L3.
Tinnitus: FA11, HN1, HN2, OFA26, OHN25, OHN29, Hand 11, K-L3, K-L17, K-L31.
Deafness: FA11, HN1, OFA22, OFA23, OFA25, OFA26, OFA27, OFA28, OHN9, OHN14, OHN15,
    OHN16, OHN21, OHN23, OHN24, OHN25, OHN29, OAR29, OAR32, OLE50, OLE51, K-L3.
Menière's Disease: K-L5, K-L15.
Vertigo: FA1, HN2, LE10, OFA7, OFA10, OHN18, OHN26, Hand 25, K-L5.
Deaf-mutism: FA11, HN1, OFA23, OFA24, OFA26, OHN20, OAR37.

CROSS-INDEX OF THE POINTS

Anmian 1	HN3	Chongjian	CA13	Fuyamen	OHN31
Anmian 2	HN4	Chuangxinmen	OCA11		
Anmian 3	ODL19	Chuchueh	ODL9	Gangmensixue	ODL57
Anmian 4	OLE65	Chuqixue	OLE75	Ganrexue	ODL14
		Cunping	OAR34	Ganshi	OCA9
Bafeng points	LE12			Ganyandian	OLE69
Bahua	ODL59	Dagukong	OAR47	Genjin	LE9
Baichongwo	OLE44	Dalun	OLE23	Genping	LE11
Bailao	HN9	Damen	OHN27	Gongzhong	AR6
Baintao	HN5	Dannangxue	LE7	Guangcai	OFA21
Baizhongfeng	ODL7	Dayan	ODL52	Guantu	OLE9
Banmen	OAR12	Dianxian	ODL27		
Baxie points	AR12	Dihe	OFA17	Haiquan	M2
Bazhuixia	ODL22	Dijia 1	OHN35	Heding	LE4
Bikong	ODL53	Dijia 2	OHN36	Hongyin	OHN3
Biliu	OFA13	Dijian	OLE62	Houcong	OHN14
Bitong	FA8	Dingchuan	DL3	Houtinggong	OHN15
Bizhong	AR7	Dingshen	OFA15	Houtingxue	OHN16
		Dingshu	OAR8	Houxuehai	OLE45
Changfeng	ODL33			Houyangguan	OLE37
Changyi	OCA22	Ehrjian	OFA20	Huanmen	ODL15
Chenggu	OLE38	Eni	OCA10	Huanyue	ODL46
Chengjian	OLE58	Erbai	AR10	Huanzhong	DL10
Chengming	OLE67	Erbeijingmaisantiao	OHN17	Huatuojiaji points	DL1
Chiqian	OHN21	Erliban	OLE48	Hubian	OAR40
Chirao	OAR31	Ezhong	OFA10	Hunshe	OCA15
Chisanxue	DL1a			Huxi	OHN11
Chixia	OHN22	Feirexue	ODL11		
Chixue	OCA2	Fengyan	OHN12	Jiabi	OFA12
Chonggu	ODL4	Fengyan	OAR18	Jiachengjiang	FA10

109

Jianei	M4	Liuhua	ODL59	Qiying	OHN5
Jianhao	AR8	Liujingzhuipang	ODL3	Qizhong	CA11
Jiankua	OLE1	Liwai	OLE49	Quanjian	OAR42
Jianming	OAR20	Longhan	OCA7	Quanshengzu	OLE78
Jianming	OFA3	Longmen	OCA25		
Jianming 1	OFA3a	Luojing	OHN10	Ronghou	OHN9
Jianming 2	OFA3b	Luolingwu	OAR39		
Jianming 3	OFA3c	Luoshang	OAR32	Sanchi	OAR25
Jianming 4	OFA3d	Luozhen	AR14	Sanliwai	OAR28
Jianming 5	ODL24			Sanshang	OAR49
Jianneiling	AR1	Maibu	LE3	Sanxiao	OFA14
Jianqian	AR2	Maigen	ODL45	Shangbafeng points	LE13
Jiantongdian	DL4	Meihua	OCA13	Shangbaxie points	AR13
Jianxi	OLE18	Mingyan	OAR46	Shangen	OFA7
Jiaoling	OLE7	Muming	OFA11	Shangergen	OHN13
Jiaoyi	OLE64	Muzhijiehengwen	OAR19	Shangfengshi	OLE12
Jiegu	ODL28	Muzhilihengwen	OLE83	Shanghouxi	OAR37
Jiehexue	ODL8			Shangjingming	OFA1
Jiejian	OLE41	Naoquing	LE10	Shanglianquan	HN6
Jifeng	ODL58	Naoshang	AR5	Shanglong	OFA23
Jingbi	HN10	Neihegu	OAR13	Shangming	FA5
Jingxia	OLE56	Neihuaijian	OLE73	Shangquchi	OAR23
Jingzhong	OHN32	Neijingming	OFA5	Shangququan	OLE46
Jingzhong	OCA17	Neiyangchi	OAR10	Shangxi	OLE71
Jinjin	M1	Neiyingxiang	OFA18	Shangxuehai	OLE43
Jisanxue	ODL1	Niushangxue	OAR30	Shangyangquan	OLE30
Jiuneifan	OLE60	Nuemen	OAR41	Shangyingxian	FA7
Jiuqi	ODL48	Nuxi	OLE79	Shaoyangwei	OLE70
Jiuwaifan 1	OLE68			Shenrexue	ODL17
Jiuwaifan 2	OLE59	Panggu	OLE80	Shenxi	OLE14
Jixia	OLE40	Panglaogong	OAR14	Shenxin	ODL37
Jubi	AR4	Panglianquan	OHN2	Shenzhou	OAR21
Jueyun	OCA19	Pangqiang	ODL55	Shenzi	DL6
Jugoxia	ODL10	Pigen	ODL31	Shezhu	M3
Juquan	M5	Pinxueling	ODL51	Shicang	OCA12
Juqueshu	ODL12	Pirexue	ODL16	Shiguan	OCA14
				Shimian	OLE87
Kuangu	OLE20	Qiabinzhong	OLE8	Shiqizhui	DL8
Kuanjiu	OLE2	Qiahoushangji	ODL40	Shiwang	OAR48
Kuiyangxue	ODL30	Qiangkua	OLE3	Shixuan	AR16
		Qiangyin	OHN7	Shoujinmen	OAR9
Lanweixue	LE6	Qianhouyinzhu	OLE85	Shouzhongping	OAR16
Liaoliao	OLE24	Qianjin	OLE11	Shubian	ODL25
Libian	ODL54	Qianzhong	FA9	Shuishang	CA2
Lijimingandian	OLE63	Qichuan	ODL18	Shuxi	CA10
Lineiting	OLE84	Qiduan	OLE88	Sifeng	AR15
Lingbao	OLE31	Qijingzhuipang	ODL5	Sili	OLE54
Linghou	LE8	Qimen	OCA21	Silian	OLE33
Lingxia	OLE50	Qisbian	OCA27	Siqiang	OLE16
Lishang	OLE47	Qiuhou	FA4	Sishencong	OHN26

110

Taijian	AR3	Xiachengshan	OLE61	Yijing	OCA20
Taiyang	FA3	Xiafutu	OHN8	Yilong	HN1
Taiyinqiao	OLE74	Xiajiaoshu	ODL56	Yiming	HN2
Tanchuan	OCA6	Xiajingming	OFA2	Yinbian	OCA26
Tanfu	OLE19	Xiajishu	ODL36	Yingshang	AR9
Tankang	OLE15	Xiakunlun	OLE77	Yingxia	OAR29
Tanli	OLE17	Xiaoerjixiong	OCA4	Yiniao	OLE66
Tianling	OAR1	Xiaogukong	OAR44	Yinkang	OLE5
Tianting	OHN23	Xiaokuai	OCA1	Yinkou	ODL20
Tiaoyue	ODL42	Xiaotianxin	OAR11	Yinshang	OLE10
Tingcong	OFA27	Xiawenliu	OAR33	Yintang	FA1
Tingling	FA11	Xiaxiabai	OAR4	Yinwai 1	OLE36
Tingling	OFA26	Xiaxinshi	OHN33	Yinwai 2	OLE35
Tinglongjian	OFA25	Xiayamen	OHN30	Yinwai 3	OLE34
Tingmin	OFA28	Xiazhongji	OCA23	Yinxia	OLE26
Tingtou	OCA24	Xiazhui	ODL49	Yishu	ODL21
Tingxiang	OFA22	Ximingxia	OHN24	Youyi	OCA8
Tingxue	OFA24	Xinfutu	OLE13	Yutian	ODL50
Tituoxue	CA6	Xingfen	OHN19	Yuwei	OFA6
Tiwei	CA1	Xingqixue	CA5	Yuyao	FA2
Tongbian	OCA16	Xinhuantiao	OLE4	Yuyue	M1
Tongerdao	OHN25	Xinleitou	OCA3		
Tongling	OAR38	Xinquchi	OAR24	Zengming 1	OFA4
Tongming	OFA9	Xinsheng	OLE42	Zengming 2	OFA4a
Tounie	OFA19	Xinshi	HN8	Zengyin	HN7
Tunzhong	ODL47	Xiongdaji	OCA5	Zequian	OAR5
Tuoguangming	OFA8	Xishang	ODL39	Zexia	OAR6
		Xishang	OAR7	Zhantan	ODL38
		Xiwai	OLE39	Zhihuanjin	OLE72
Waidingchuan	ODL6	Xixia	OLE25	Zhili	OLE27
Waierdaokou	OHN29	Xiyan points	LE5	Zhinao	ODL2
Waihuaijian	OLE76	Xuechou	ODL32	Zhiou	OHN4
Waijinjin	OHN1	Xuefu	ODL34	Zhiping	OLE81
Waiming	FA6	Xueyadian	DL2	Zhitan 1	OAR3
Waisiman	OCA18	Xutse	DL1b	Zhitan 6	OLE55
Waiyuye	OHN1			Zhiwen	OLE82
Waizhili	OLE28	Yaming	OHN20	Zhixie	CA8
Wanli	OLE52	Yanchi	OHN18	Zhiyang	OAR22
Weibao	CA7	Yangkang	OLE6	Zhizhang	OAR17
Weiguanxiashu	ODL23	Yankou	OFA16	Zhongjiaoshu	ODL29
Weilei	CA3	Yaogan	ODL44	Zhongjie	OHN28
Weirexue	ODL13	Yaoqi	DL9	Zhongkong	ODL43
Weishang	OLE29	Yaotang (1, 2 & 3)	OAR36	Zhongkui	OAR45
Weishangxue	CA4	Yaoyan	DL7	Zhongquan	AR11
Weishu	DL5	Yaoyi	ODL41	Zhongquan	OAR35
Weixia	OLE57	Yatong	AR17	Zhoujian	OAR26
Weiyinlian	LE2	Yatong	OAR15	Zhoushu	OAR27
Wuhu	OAR43	Yaxue	OHN6	Zhuding	OFA29
Wuling	OLE32	Yeling	OAR2	Zhuoyu	ODL26
Wuming	DL11	Yeniao	CA12	Zhuzhang	ODL35

Zigong	CA9	Zuogu	LE1	Zuyicong	OLE51
Zuluo	OLE21	Zuoyi	OCA8	Zuzhongping	OLE53
Zuming	OLE22	Zuxin	OLE86		